Enoc Hernández

Health Care Ethics

Enoc Hernández

Health Care Ethics

Fundamentals for an Integral and Proactive Approach

ScienciaScripts

Cover image: www.ingimage.com

This book is a translation from the original published under ISBN 978-613-9-40449-0.

Publisher:
Sciencia Scripts
is a trademark of
Dodo Books Indian Ocean Ltd. and OmniScriptum S.R.L publishing group

120 High Road, East Finchley, London, N2 9ED, United Kingdom
Str. Armeneasca 28/1, office 1, Chisinau MD-2012, Republic of Moldova, Europe
Printed at: see last page
ISBN: 978-620-7-68719-0

TITLE: HEALTH CARE ETHICS
SUBTITLE: FUNDAMENTALS FOR A COMPREHENSIVE AND PROACTIVE APPROACH
AUTHOR: ENOC ISAÍ HERNÁNDEZ CANTÚ

FOREWORD

Health is a fundamental human right and an essential pillar for the well-being and sustainable development of societies. However, despite remarkable advances in medicine and technology, we persist in facing significant challenges that require a comprehensive, ethical and proactive approach. "Health Care Ethics: Foundations for a Comprehensive and Proactive Approach" is a work that addresses these challenges with a multidimensional perspective, offering a comprehensive guide for health professionals, academics and anyone committed to improving global wellbeing.The origin of this book lies in the conviction that health care begins with the individual, but must be supported by an equitable and accessible health system. The main thesis is based on the "Health Decalogue for the 21st Century: A Global Call to Action", a set of principles that promotes holistic awareness, prevention, empowerment, equity, innovation, education, intersectoral collaboration, sustainability, ethics and global solidarity.Each chapter of this book has been carefully developed to provide both a theoretical framework and practical strategies that can be implemented in a variety of contexts. From health promotion and self-care to the adoption of advanced technologies and cross-sector collaboration, this book offers a holistic approach that recognises the interconnectedness of physical, mental, emotional and social factors that influence health.The relevance of this work is reinforced by recent global events, such as the COVID-19 pandemic, which have highlighted the importance of resilient health systems and the need for international cooperation. These challenges have revealed existing inequalities and the urgency of adopting an ethical and human rights-based approach to ensure that everyone has access to the health care they need. The chapter on holistic awareness reminds us that health cannot be fragmented; it is a dynamic and multidimensional state that must be addressed in its entirety. Prevention and self-care are the cornerstone of a sustainable health system, and the empowerment of individuals and communities is crucial for effective health management. Equity and universal access are essential principles that must guide our policies and practices, ensuring that no one is left behind.Innovation and technology in the service of health have the potential to transform health care, but they must be integrated in an ethical and equitable manner. Education and health literacy empower people to make informed choices, and intersectoral collaboration is vital to address the social determinants of health. Sustainability and resilience in global health ensure that our health systems can meet present and future challenges, while ethics and human rights are the foundation on which all our actions and policies must be built. Finally, global action and solidarity are essential to address health challenges that transcend borders. In an interconnected world, international cooperation and collaboration are essential to improve global health and well-being. This book is not only a call to action, but also a practical guide for those committed to improving health and well-being. I hope that "Health Care Ethics: Foundations for a Comprehensive and Proactive Approach" will inspire health professionals and all readers to adopt a more comprehensive, ethical and proactive approach in their daily practice, and to work together to build a healthier and more equitable future for all.

Enoc Isaí Hernández Cantú

May 2024

CONTENT

INTRODUCTION

Health as an Individual and Collective Responsibility

Health is one of the fundamental pillars on which the well-being of individuals and societies is built. In an interconnected and ever-changing world, health promotion has emerged as an essential priority to ensure quality of life. Despite significant advances in medicine and technology, health remains a global challenge that requires a comprehensive and proactive approach.

Health care ethics is a philosophy that recognises that wellbeing begins with the individual and extends to the community and the world at large. This book, "Health Care Ethics: Foundations for a Comprehensive and Proactive Approach", explores how ethical principles and core values can guide our actions and decisions in health care. It is intended for health professionals, academics, students and anyone interested in understanding and applying an ethical approach to health care.

Health as a Dynamic and Multidimensional State

We start from the premise that health is a dynamic and multidimensional state, influenced by physical, mental, emotional and social factors. This holistic approach recognises that health is not simply the absence of disease, but a state of complete wellbeing that must be nurtured and protected. We recognise the importance of developing a holistic awareness of wellness and taking proactive action for its preservation and constant improvement. This approach is articulated in the "Health Decalogue for the 21st Century: A Global Call to Action", which provides clear and practical guidance for promoting health and wellness at the individual and collective levels.

Global Health Context

Today's health challenges are more complex than ever. Chronic diseases, pandemics, inequalities in access to services and the effects of climate change are just some of the problems we face. These challenges require innovative and collaborative solutions that transcend national borders and sectors of society. Global health has become a central issue on the international agenda, and it is imperative that we take an ethical and caring approach to addressing these problems.

The 21st Century Health Decalogue

One of the main proposals of this book is the "Health Decalogue for the 21st Century: A Call to Global Action". This Decalogue is based on a profound reflection on the current challenges and opportunities in the field of health, offering a practical and ethical guide for the promotion of holistic wellbeing. Each of the principles, presented below, seeks to inspire and guide individuals, communities and health professionals in their quest for a healthier and more equitable future.

1. Integral Awareness: Health is a dynamic and multidimensional state, influenced by physical, mental, emotional and social factors. It promotes the development of a holistic awareness of well-being and encourages proactive action for its preservation and constant improvement.

2. Prevention and Self-Care: Prevention is prioritised as the cornerstone of health. A proactive approach to self-care is encouraged, consciously anticipating and mitigating health risks through healthy lifestyles and informed choices.

3. Individual and Collective Empowerment: Each individual has the power and responsibility to take care of their own health. It promotes the empowerment of individuals in the management of their wellbeing, as well as the support and strengthening of communities in their pursuit of health and wellbeing.

4. Equity and Universal Access: Equity in access to health services and resources needed to maintain and improve health is promoted.

It advocates for health systems that are inclusive and accessible to all, regardless of ethnicity, gender, sexual orientation, socio-economic status or geographic location.

5. Innovation and Technology for Health: The transformative potential of innovation and technology in health is recognised. It encourages the development and adoption of innovative solutions that improve access, efficiency and quality of health care in all communities.

6. Health Education and Literacy: Health education and literacy are valued as essential tools to empower people to make informed decisions about their well-being. Health education is promoted from an early age and provides accurate and accessible information on health issues.

7. Intersectoral Collaboration: Health is recognised as an outcome of actions that transcend the boundaries of the health sector. Intersectoral collaboration between governments, organisations, businesses and civil society is encouraged to address the social determinants of health and promote healthy environments.

8. Sustainability and Resilience: Health is valued as a precious resource that must be protected and preserved for present and future generations. It promotes sustainable practices that promote the health of the planet and builds resilience to environmental and climatic challenges that affect our health.

9. Ethics and Human Rights: Health is recognised as a fundamental human right and an ethical imperative. Human rights are protected and promoted in all health-related actions, ensuring equity, dignity and respect for all people.

10. Global Action and Solidarity: It is recognised that health is a global issue that requires a coordinated and solidarity-based response at the international level. It is works as a global community to address the most pressing health challenges and promote a healthier and more equitable world for all.

Objectives of the book

This book has several fundamental objectives:

- Provide practical guidance: To offer health professionals practical guidance based on ethical principles and core values to improve the quality of health care.

- Raise awareness: Raise awareness of the importance of a holistic and proactive approach to health, including prevention, self-care and empowerment.

- Promote equity: Advocate for equity and universal access to health services, highlighting the importance of inclusive and accessible health systems.

- Driving innovation: Highlighting the role of innovation and technology in transforming healthcare and improving global health.

- Facilitating collaboration: Encourage intersectoral collaboration to address the social determinants of health and promote healthy environments.

In the following chapters, we will explore each of these issues in detail, providing both a theoretical framework and practical examples and case studies that illustrate how these principles can be applied in everyday practice.

CHAPTER 1

INTEGRAL CONSCIOUSNESS: A HOLISTIC APPROACH TO WELL-BEING

INTRODUCTION TO INTEGRAL CONSCIOUSNESS

Health, in its broadest sense, is much more than the absence of disease. It is a state of complete physical, mental and social well-being. This definition, proposed by the World Health Organisation (WHO), reflects the complexity and multidimensionality of human well-being. In this context, holistic awareness emerges as a necessary approach to address health holistically. This approach recognises that health cannot be adequately understood and promoted if it is limited to only one aspect of the human being.Integral awareness is a state of deep perception and understanding of all the factors that influence our health. It includes self-awareness of our own physical, emotional, mental and social needs, as well as an understanding of how these dimensions interact and affect each other. Adopting a holistic awareness approach means recognising that wellness is a dynamic state that requires constant effort and proactive attention.

The Components of Integral Consciousness

1. Physical Well-being

Physical well-being is the most tangible component and often the easiest to identify. It includes aspects such as nutrition, exercise, sleep and disease prevention. Holistic awareness in this area involves not only maintaining a disease-free body, but also optimising our physical capacity through healthy habits. This includes a balanced diet, regular physical activity, and proper management of rest and sleep.

2. Mental and Emotional Well-being

Mental and emotional health is just as crucial as physical health. Holistic awareness in this regard involves recognising and managing our emotions, thoughts and behaviours. It includes practices such as meditation, mindfulness and psychotherapy, which help us to maintain mental and emotional balance. In addition, it is essential to develop resilience, the ability to adapt and recover from adversity.

3. Social Welfare

Human beings are inherently social. Our relationships and connections with others play a crucial role in our health and well-being. Holistic awareness of social well-being involves cultivating healthy relationships, establishing a strong support network and actively participating in the community. It also means being aware of how our interactions and relationships affect our overall well-being and that of others.

4. Spiritual Wellbeing

Spiritual well-being may be a more subjective dimension, but it is no less important. It involves a sense of purpose and meaning in life, as well as the beliefs and values that guide our actions. Integral awareness in this regard may include practices such as meditation, prayer, or any activity that promotes a sense of connection to something greater than oneself.

Integration of the Components of Well-being

Adopting a holistic awareness approach requires the integration of these four components. It is not a matter of addressing each in isolation, but of recognising how they interrelate and influence each other. For example, emotional stress can manifest itself in physical symptoms, such as headaches or digestive problems. Similarly, poor nutrition can affect our mental and emotional ability to handle stress.

Practices for Developing Integral Consciousness

1. Regular Self-Assessment

Regular self-assessment is a fundamental practice in developing holistic awareness. This can include keeping a health diary, recording eating habits, sleep patterns, physical activity levels and emotional states. Reflecting on these observations allows us to identify patterns and areas that need attention.

2. Mindfulness and Meditation

Mindfulness practice and meditation are powerful tools for increasing self-awareness and holistic well-being. These practices help us to be present in the moment, to recognise and accept our thoughts and emotions without judgement, and to reduce stress and anxiety.

3. Continuing Education

Staying informed about health and wellness issues is essential for holistic awareness. This can include reading books, attending workshops or courses, and following health and wellness experts. Continuing education provides us with the tools and knowledge we need to make informed decisions about our health.

4. Connecting with the Community

Participating in community activities and cultivating meaningful relationships are key aspects of social well-being. This may include joining support groups, participating in community events, or simply spending quality time with friends and family.

Challenges and Barriers to Integral Consciousness

1. Modern Lifestyles

Modern lifestyles, often characterised by stress, lack of time and information overload, can be significant barriers to the development of holistic awareness. The culture of rushing and multitasking takes time away from reflecting on our health and well-being.

2. Lack of Education and Resources

In many communities, lack of education and resources on holistic health issues can be a barrier. It is crucial to promote educational programmes and provide access to resources that support holistic wellness.

3. Stigma and Social Perception

The stigma associated with mental and emotional health can prevent people from seeking the help they need. Changing social perceptions about these issues is vital to encourage a holistic approach to health.

Conclusion

Integrative mindfulness is a holistic approach that recognises the complexity of human wellbeing and aligns closely with ethical principles of healthcare. By integrating the physical, mental, emotional, social and spiritual components, we not only develop a deeper and more proactive understanding of our health, but also act in accordance with an ethical framework that values and respects the whole human being. From an ethical perspective, holistic awareness promotes the dignity and autonomy of individuals by recognising the interdependence of the different dimensions of well-being. This holistic approach facilitates informed and responsible decision-making about our well-being, which is an act of respect for our own autonomy and dignity. Furthermore, promoting holistic awareness has significant ethical implications in terms of equity and social justice. By advocating an approach that considers all dimensions of wellbeing, we are recognising and valuing the diversity of people's experiences and needs. This includes the ethical responsibility of health professionals to provide care that is inclusive, holistic and person-centred.The ethics of healthcare urges us to look beyond physical symptoms and consider health in its totality, including mental, emotional, social and spiritual aspects. In doing so, we not only improve our quality of life, but also empower people to make informed and responsible decisions about their well-being, respecting their dignity and autonomy.

CHAPTER 2

PREVENTION AND SELF-CARE: THE CORNERSTONE OF HEALTH INTRODUCTION TO PREVENTION AND SELF-CARE

Prevention and self-care are the cornerstones of maintaining and improving our health throughout our lives. Rather than reacting to illness, prevention and self-care invite us to take a proactive approach, anticipating health problems before they occur. This approach is not only more effective in terms of health, but also more sustainable and cost-effective for health systems and communities.

Prevention and self-care are based on the idea that each individual has the responsibility and power to manage his or her own health. This involves adopting healthy habits, having regular medical check-ups and being informed about risks and preventive measures. In this chapter, we will explore the key principles of prevention and self-care, and provide practical strategies for incorporating them into everyday life.

The Principles of Prevention

1. Primary Prevention

Primary prevention focuses on preventing the development of diseases and health conditions before they occur. This includes:

• Vaccination: Vaccines are a fundamental tool for preventing infectious diseases. Adequate immunisation can eradicate diseases and significantly reduce their prevalence in the population.

• Healthy Lifestyles: Adopt a balanced diet, engage in regular physical activity, avoid smoking and moderate alcohol consumption. These habits help to strengthen the immune system and prevent chronic diseases.

• Education and Awareness: Informing people about health risks and preventive measures they can take. Education

Health education should start from an early age and continue throughout life.

2. Secondary Prevention

Secondary prevention involves the early detection and timely treatment of incipient diseases to prevent their progression. This includes:

• Regular Health Exams: Get regular medical check-ups and screening tests such as mammograms, colonoscopies and blood tests. These tests can identify health problems at an earlier stage, when they are more treatable.

• Early Detection: Identify and treat risk factors such as hypertension, high cholesterol and overweight. Early intervention can prevent serious complications and improve long-term health outcomes.

3. Tertiary Prevention

Tertiary prevention focuses on reducing complications and improving the quality of life of people who already have a chronic disease. This includes:

• Rehabilitation: Physical and mental rehabilitation programmes for patients with chronic diseases or disabilities. These programmes help patients to regain function and improve their quality of life.

• Chronic Disease Management: Controlling conditions such as diabetes, hypertension and heart disease through medication, lifestyle changes and continuous monitoring. Effective chronic disease management can prevent disease progression and reduce the risk of complications.

Self-care strategies

1. Healthy Eating

A balanced diet is essential for maintaining good health. Healthy eating includes:

• Nutrient Variety: Consume a wide variety of foods to get all the nutrients you need. A diet rich in fruits, vegetables, lean proteins and whole grains provides a solid foundation for health.

• Portion Control: Be mindful of portions to avoid overweight and obesity. Overeating can lead to a number of health problems, including heart disease and diabetes.

• Hydration: Drink enough water daily. Adequate hydration is crucial to maintain bodily functions and prevent dehydration.

• Limit Processed Foods: Reduce consumption of foods high in sugars, saturated fats and sodium. Processed foods often contain unhealthy ingredients that can contribute to chronic diseases.

2. Regular Physical Activity

Regular exercise is crucial for maintaining physical and mental health. Recommendations include:

• Aerobic Exercise: At least 150 minutes of moderate aerobic activity or 75 minutes of intense activity per week. Activities such as walking, running, swimming or cycling are excellent choices.

• Muscle Strengthening: Perform muscle-strengthening exercises at least two days a week. These exercises can include weight lifting, yoga or Pilates.

• Flexibility and Balance: Incorporate stretching and balance exercises, especially for older adults. These exercises help prevent falls and maintain mobility.

3. Stress Management

Chronic stress can have negative effects on health. Strategies to manage stress include:

• Mindfulness and Meditation: Practising mindfulness and meditation to reduce stress. These practices help to calm the mind and improve concentration.

• Leisure Time: Make time for recreational activities and hobbies. Engaging in activities that we enjoy can improve our mood and reduce stress.

• Relaxation Techniques: Use deep breathing techniques, yoga and other forms of relaxation. These techniques can help relieve tension and promote a state of calm.

4. Quality Dream

Adequate sleep is essential for overall health. Recommendations for improving sleep quality include:

• Sleep Routine: Maintain a regular sleep schedule, even on weekends. Going to bed and waking up at the same time every day helps regulate the biological clock.

• Sleep Friendly Environment: Create a dark, quiet and cool environment for sleeping. A comfortable environment can improve the quality of sleep.

• Avoid stimulants: Limit caffeine intake and avoid using electronic devices before bedtime. Blue light from screens can interfere with melatonin production and make it difficult to sleep.

5. Personal Hygiene

Proper personal hygiene helps prevent disease and maintain overall health. It includes:

• Dental hygiene: Brush teeth at least twice a day and floss daily. Proper dental hygiene prevents gum disease and tooth decay.

• Body hygiene: Bathe regularly and wash hands frequently. Maintaining good body hygiene is essential to prevent infection.

• Skin Care: Protect skin from the sun and keep it moisturised. Using sunscreen and moisturising lotions helps to maintain skin health.

Benefits of Prevention and Self-Care

1. Disease Reduction

The adoption of preventive and self-care habits significantly reduces the risk of developing chronic diseases such as diabetes, heart disease and cancer. Effective prevention can improve public health and reduce the burden on health systems.

2. Improving Quality of Life

People who practice self-care tend to have a better quality of life, with more energy, better mood and lower incidence of disease. A proactive approach to health can increase longevity and overall well-being.

3. Economic Savings

Prevention and self-care can reduce health care costs by reducing the need for expensive treatments and hospitalisations. Investing in preventive health can generate significant savings for both individuals and health systems.

Challenges and Barriers to Prevention and Self-Care

1. Lack of Time and Motivation

Many people find it difficult to find the time and motivation to adopt healthy habits due to busy and stressful lifestyles. Health promotion should include strategies to motivate and support people to adopt healthy practices.

2. Access to Resources

Lack of access to resources such as healthy foods, safe places to exercise and health services can be a significant barrier. It is critical to work to improve the accessibility and availability of health resources in all communities.

3. Information and Education

Lack of accurate information and education about the importance of prevention and self-care can prevent people from adopting these habits. Health education must be a priority to provide people with the knowledge and tools they need to manage their health.

Conclusion

Prevention and self-care are essential to maintaining and improving our health and are closely linked to the ethical principles of health care. Adopting a proactive approach, based on primary, secondary and tertiary prevention and self-care practices, not only allows us to live a healthier life, but also to live a healthier life. healthier and more fulfilling lives, but also reflects an ethical commitment to our own health and that of our community. From an ethical perspective, prevention and self-care respect and promote people's autonomy and dignity by providing them with the tools and knowledge to make informed decisions about their well-being. This approach also underlines the importance of personal and collective responsibility in health promotion.In addition, promoting prevention and self-care has a strong social justice and equity component. Ensuring that all people have access to the information, resources and support they need to prevent disease and manage their health is an ethical imperative. This includes overcoming socio-economic, cultural and educational barriers that prevent some people from adopting healthy habits and engaging in preventive practices. Health professionals have an ethical responsibility to promote prevention and self-care by providing education, support and resources to all people, regardless of their socio-economic or cultural background. In doing so, they contribute to reducing health inequalities and promoting a holistic approach that benefits both individuals and communities.

CHAPTER 3

INDIVIDUAL AND COLLECTIVE EMPOWERMENT IN HEALTH MANAGEMENT

Introduction to Health Empowerment

Health empowerment refers to the process by which people acquire the knowledge, skills and confidence to make informed and responsible decisions about their own health. This concept is central to the promotion of health and wellbeing, as it recognises the capacity and responsibility of each individual to manage their health. Furthermore, empowerment applies not only at the individual level, but also at the community level, where collaboration and mutual support can amplify the benefits of personal empowerment.

Health empowerment is a key factor in achieving optimal health. It involves not only the acquisition of information, but also the ability to use that information to make informed decisions and take control of one's own health. Education, training and skills development are essential elements of this process. In this chapter, we will delve into the key concepts and strategies of individual and collective empowerment, providing practical guidance for applying them in daily life and in the community.

Individual Empowerment: Concepts and Strategies

1. Knowledge Acquisition

Knowledge is the first step towards empowerment. People need to be well informed about their health conditions, treatment options and preventive measures. This includes:

• Health Education: Educational programmes that provide accurate and accessible information on relevant health issues. These programmes should be ongoing and tailored to the needs of different population groups.

• Access to Information: Availability of reliable resources such as health websites, books, brochures and mobile apps. Information should be easy to understand and applicable in everyday life.

• Ongoing training: Participation in workshops, courses and seminars on health and wellbeing. Training should focus on practical skills that people can use to manage their health.

2. Skills Development

Knowledge without practical skills has limited impact. People must learn to apply what they know in their daily lives. This includes:

• Disease self-management: Skills to monitor and manage chronic conditions such as diabetes or hypertension. This may include self-monitoring of blood sugar levels, blood pressure and adherence to treatment plans.

• Decision-making: Skills to evaluate treatment options and make informed decisions. This includes the ability to understand the benefits and risks of different treatments and to make decisions based on personal values and preferences.

• Effective Communication: Skills to communicate effectively with health professionals and express your needs and concerns. Clear and open communication is crucial to receiving the best possible care.

3. Confidence Building

Self-confidence is crucial to the successful implementation of health practices. Strategies to build confidence include:

• Psychological support: Therapies and support groups that reinforce self-esteem and self-confidence. Emotional support is essential for coping with health challenges.

• Gradual Successes: Setting achievable health goals and celebrating successes. Recognising and celebrating small successes can motivate people to continue their self-care efforts.

• Role Models: Examples of people who have successfully managed their health and can serve as inspiration. Testimonials and success stories can motivate others to take similar steps.

Collective Empowerment: Building Healthy Communities

Collective empowerment involves collaboration and mutual support within a community to improve the health of all its members. This approach recognises that an individual's health is interconnected with the health of their community.

1. Support Networks

Support networks are fundamental to collective empowerment. These may include:

• Support groups: Spaces where people can share experiences, offer and receive emotional support. Support groups can be face-to-face or virtual, and should be accessible to all members of the community.

• Social Networking: Using digital platforms to create online communities of support. Social networks can connect people with similar interests and challenges, facilitating the exchange of information and support.

• Family and Friends: Encourage mutual support within close circles. Strong personal relationships can provide crucial emotional support in times of need.

2. Community Education

Community education promotes collective health through the dissemination of knowledge and healthy practices. This includes:

• Talks and Workshops: Organise educational events on health issues relevant to the community. These events should be interactive and accessible to all members of the community.

• Awareness campaigns: Initiatives to inform and sensitise the community about health risks and preventive measures. Campaigns can use a variety of media, from leaflets to social media.

• Collaboration with Schools and Organisations: Partnerships with local institutions to promote health education. Schools and community organisations can play a key role in health education, reaching a wide audience.

3. Participation and Community Action

Active community participation in health promotion is essential. Strategies to encourage this participation include:

• Community projects: Initiatives such as community gardens, group exercise programmes and health fairs. These projects can improve the physical and mental health of participants, as well as strengthen community cohesion.

• Volunteering: Encourage volunteering in health and wellness-related activities. Volunteering can provide a sense of purpose and belonging, as well as improve community health.

• Advocacy and Health Policy: Involvement in policy advocacy to promote health equity and access to health services. Advocacy may include lobbying, lobbying, lobbying and advocacy.

collaboration with legislators and the promotion of inclusive health policies.

Health Empowerment Benefits

1. Improving Health and Wellbeing

Individual and collective empowerment leads to better health outcomes. Empowered people are more likely to adopt healthy habits, comply with medical treatment and participate in preventive activities. Active participation in health management can improve both physical and mental health.

2. Reducing Health Inequalities

Empowerment can help reduce health inequalities by providing all people, regardless of their socio-economic status, with the knowledge and tools to manage their health. Education and accessible resources are essential to level the playing field.

3. Community Strengthening

Empowered communities are more resilient and able to address health challenges collectively. This strengthens social cohesion and a sense of belonging, creating a healthier and more supportive environment for all.

Challenges and Barriers to Empowerment

1. Access to Information and Resources

Lack of access to reliable information and adequate resources can be a significant barrier to empowerment. Improving the availability and accessibility of these resources is essential. Technology and community libraries can play a crucial role in this area.

2. Cultural and Social Barriers

Cultural and social norms can influence health-related perception and behaviour. Overcoming these barriers requires culturally sensitive and adapted approaches. Collaboration with community leaders and cultural organisations can facilitate acceptance and implementation of healthy practices.

3. Socio-economic inequalities

Socio-economic inequalities can limit opportunities for empowerment. Addressing these inequalities is crucial to ensure that everyone has the opportunity to manage their health effectively. Inclusive policies and assistance programmes can help reduce these disparities.

Strategies for Promoting Empowerment

1. Inclusive Health Policies

Develop and promote health policies that are inclusive and support the empowerment of all people, especially those in vulnerable situations. Policies should focus on equity and accessibility, ensuring that everyone has access to necessary health care and resources.

2. Education and Training Programmes

Implement education and training programmes that provide people with the knowledge and skills necessary to manage their health. These programmes should be ongoing and tailored to the needs of the community, using participatory and interactive teaching methods.

3. Strengthening Support Networks

Encourage and support the creation of community support networks that facilitate collective empowerment. Support networks may include groups of support, community organisations and online platforms that connect people with similar interests and challenges.

Conclusion

Individual and collective empowerment is essential for effective health management and is deeply linked to the ethical principles of health care. From an ethical perspective, empowering people means respecting their autonomy, dignity and ability to make informed decisions about their well-being. By acquiring knowledge, developing skills and building confidence, people can take control of their health and well-being, which is an act of respect for their autonomy and dignity.In addition, collective empowerment reinforces social justice and equity, fundamental principles in the ethics of health care. By strengthening communities and promoting collaboration and mutual support, it fosters an environment in which all members have equal access to resources and opportunities to maintain and improve their health. This not only improves the quality of life for individuals, but also strengthens community cohesion and resilience, reflecting an ethical commitment to collective well-being. Empowerment in health also implies an ethical responsibility on the part of health professionals to provide accurate information, support skills development and create an environment of trust and respect. Health professionals must act as facilitators of empowerment, promoting equity and ensuring that all people, regardless of socio-economic or cultural status, have the opportunity to manage their health effectively.

CHAPTER 4

EQUITY AND UNIVERSAL ACCESS TO HEALTH SERVICES INTRODUCTION TO HEALTH EQUITY

Health equity is a fundamental principle that seeks to ensure that all people have an equal opportunity to reach their full health potential, regardless of their social, economic or cultural background. Health equity focuses not only on equal access to health services, but also on the elimination of barriers that prevent certain populations from receiving quality care. Universal access to health services is a goal that many health systems around the world have set out to achieve. This concept implies that all people, regardless of their economic or geographic situation, should be able to access the health services they need without facing financial barriers. In this chapter, we explore the key concepts of equity and universal access in health, the barriers that exist, and strategies for overcoming these challenges.

Key Concepts of Equity and Universal Access

1. Health Equity

Equity in health implies that all individuals have a fair and equal opportunity to be healthy. This implies:

• Fair Distribution of Resources: Health resources should be distributed equitably, ensuring that vulnerable populations receive the necessary support.

• Elimination of Inequalities: Health inequalities caused by social, economic and environmental factors must be identified and eliminated.

• Social Justice: Equity in health is intrinsically linked to social justice, where fair and equitable treatment for all people is advocated.

2. Universal Access to Health Services

Universal access to health services refers to the availability of essential health services to all, without financial barriers or discrimination. This includes:

• Comprehensive coverage: Providing a wide range of health services, from prevention and treatment to rehabilitation and palliative care.

• Financial Accessibility: Ensuring that the costs of health services are not a barrier to receiving care.

• Geographic Availability: Ensure that health services are available and accessible in all regions, including rural and remote areas.

• Quality of Services: Ensure that health services are of high quality and meet professional and ethical standards.

Barriers to Equity and Universal Access

1. Economic Barriers

Economic barriers are one of the main causes of inequity in access to health services. These include:

• Direct costs: The costs of health services, such as consultations, medicines and hospitalisation, can be prohibitive for many people.

• Indirect costs: Associated costs such as transport, loss of income due to time not worked and child care.

2. Geographical Barriers

Geographic location can significantly affect access to health services. This includes:

• Inequitable Distribution of Services: Rural and remote areas often lack adequate health services.

• Distance and Transport: Distance to health centres and lack of transport can make access difficult.

3. Cultural and Social Barriers

Cultural and social barriers can limit access to health care, including:

• Language and Communication: Language differences and lack of interpretation services can be major obstacles.

• Stigmatisation and Discrimination: Discrimination based on gender, race, sexual orientation and other factors can prevent people from seeking and receiving appropriate care.

4. Health System Barriers

Health systems themselves may have structural barriers that affect equity and access, such as:

• Limited Capacity and Resources: Lack of infrastructure, staff and medical supplies.

• Inadequate Policies and Regulations: Health policies that do not adequately address the needs of all populations.

Strategies for Promoting Equity and Universal Access

1. Health Financing Reforms

To overcome economic barriers, health financing reform is essential. This includes:

• Universal Health Coverage: Implement universal health insurance systems that cover the entire population.

• Subsidies and Financial Aid: Provide subsidies and financial aid for the most vulnerable groups.

2. Improving Health Infrastructure

To address geographic barriers, health infrastructures must be improved, including:

• Construction and Maintenance of Health Centres: Ensure that there are well-equipped and maintained health centres in all areas, including rural areas.

• Health Transport Systems: Implement accessible and affordable transport systems to facilitate access to health services.

3. Training and Awareness Programmes

To overcome cultural and social barriers, training and awareness-raising programmes should be implemented, such as:

• Cultural Competence Training: Train health professionals in cultural competence to improve communication and care.

• Awareness Campaigns: Conduct campaigns to combat stigma and discrimination in health care.

4. Health System Strengthening

To remove health system barriers, it is essential to strengthen health systems, including:

• Increasing Resources and Staffing: Ensure that health facilities are adequately staffed and resourced.

• Policy Reforms: Develop and implement health policies that promote equity and universal access.

Success Stories in Equity and Universal Access

1. UK National Health System (NHS)

The National Health Service (NHS) in the UK is a flagship example of a health system that provides universal access to high quality services. Founded in 1948, the NHS is funded primarily through general taxation, enabling all UK residents to have access to free medical care at the point of use. The NHS is based on the principles of universality, equity and efficiency. It provides a wide range of services, including primary care, specialised care, hospitalisation, medicines and mental health services. In addition, the NHS has implemented specific programmes to address health inequalities, such as the NHS Health Check initiative, which offers free health checks to prevent cardiovascular disease in people aged 40-74.

The NHS has also developed referral and care coordination systems to ensure that patients receive the right services at the right time. Its funding and organisational structure allows for an equitable redistribution of resources, ensuring that areas of greatest need receive the necessary support.

2. Popular Insurance Programme in Mexico

Seguro Popular was an innovative programme in Mexico, designed to provide health coverage to people who were not covered by traditional social security. Launched in 2004, this programme sought to reduce financial barriers to accessing health care, especially for the most vulnerable populations.

Seguro Popular covered a wide range of services, from primary and preventive care to hospitalisation and specialised treatment. Financed by a combination of federal and state resources, the programme allowed families to register and receive medical care free of charge at the point of use. One of the major achievements of Seguro Popular was the significant decrease in out-of-pocket health costs for Mexican families, which reduced medical poverty. In addition, the programme improved access to health services in rural and marginalised areas by building and equipping new health units and training medical professionals.

Although Seguro Popular was replaced in 2020 by the Instituto de Salud para el Bienestar (INSABI), its legacy lives on as a model of how public health programmes can reduce inequalities and improve access to health care for all.

3. Salud en el Barrio in Brazil

The "Health in the Neighbourhood" programme (Programa Saúde da Família) in Brazil is an outstanding example of a primary care strategy that brings health services directly to disadvantaged communities. Initiated in the 1990s, the programme focuses on prevention and comprehensive care through family health teams, which include doctors, nurses, nurses' aides and community health workers. These teams work in specific geographic areas and regularly visit families in their homes, providing preventive medical care, health education and ongoing monitoring of chronic conditions. This approach allows for early and personalised intervention, tailored to the specific needs of each community.The programme has had a significant impact on reducing infant and maternal mortality rates, as well as reducing infectious and chronic diseases. Proximity and trust between health teams and the community have been key to the programme's success, promoting adherence to treatment and empowering people to manage their own health. In addition, "Health in the Neighbourhood" has strengthened the capacity of the Brazilian health system to respond to emergencies and epidemic outbreaks, demonstrating the effectiveness of primary care as the foundation of a resilient and equitable health system.

Conclusion

Equity and universal access to health services are essential goals to ensure that all people can reach their full health potential and are deeply rooted in the ethical principles of health care. From an ethical perspective, health equity requires health systems to recognise and address inequities that prevent certain groups from accessing quality care. This commitment to social justice and equity ensures that all people, regardless of socioeconomic or geographic status, receive fair treatment and access to the resources necessary for their well-being. Universal access is not only about availability, but also about ensuring that health services are accessible, affordable and culturally appropriate for all people. The ethics of health care compel us to remove barriers to access and to work towards an inclusive health system that respects and promotes the dignity of every individual.

CHAPTER 5

INNOVATION AND TECHNOLOGY FOR HEALTH INTRODUCTION TO INNOVATION AND TECHNOLOGY IN HEALTH

In today's world, innovation and technology play a crucial role in transforming healthcare and improving health outcomes. From advances in biotechnology to the use of artificial intelligence (AI) in diagnostics, technology is redefining the way we understand, prevent and treat disease. This chapter explores how technological innovations are serving health, improving access, quality and efficiency in healthcare.

Technological Advances in Diagnosis and Treatment

1. Diagnostic Imaging

Diagnostic imaging technology has advanced significantly, allowing earlier and more accurate detection of diseases. This includes:

• Magnetic Resonance Imaging (MRI) and Computed Tomography (CT): These technologies provide detailed images of the body, helping doctors identify problems that are not visible on conventional X-rays. MRI uses magnetic fields and radio waves to create detailed images of internal organs and tissues, while CT combines multiple X-ray images to generate a cross-sectional image of the body.

• High Resolution Ultrasound: Used to evaluate organs and tissues in real time, improving prenatal diagnosis and tumour detection. Advanced ultrasound allows accurate visualisation of foetuses during pregnancy and can detect congenital anomalies early.

• Molecular Imaging and PET: These allow the visualisation of biological processes at the molecular level, facilitating the diagnosis of diseases such as cancer and neurological diseases. Positron emission tomography (PET) uses radioactive tracers to observe metabolic activity in the body, helping to detect and monitor cancers, heart disease and brain disorders.

2. Artificial Intelligence and Machine Learning

Artificial intelligence (AI) and machine learning are revolutionising the field of medical diagnostics:

• AI-assisted diagnostics: Algorithms that can analyse medical images, such as X-rays and mammograms, to detect abnormalities with high accuracy. These systems can identify early signs of disease that might go unnoticed by doctors, improving diagnostic accuracy.

• Disease Prediction: AI models that analyse health data to predict the risk of diseases such as diabetes and heart disease, enabling early interventions. These models use large volumes of data to identify patterns and risk factors, enabling more proactive healthcare.

• Patient Management: Systems that use AI to optimise hospital bed management and predict resource needs. These systems can improve operational efficiency and ensure that medical resources are used effectively.

3. Personalised Therapies

Personalised medicine uses patients' genetic and molecular information to develop tailor-made treatments:

- Gene therapy: Interventions that correct genetic defects underlying certain diseases. These therapies can modify a person's genes to treat or prevent inherited diseases.
- Precision Medicine: Use of genetic profiling to personalise drug treatments, improving efficacy and reducing side effects. Treatments are designed specifically for the patient's genetic characteristics, which increases the probability of success and minimises risks.
- Immunotherapy: Treatments that use a patient's own immune system to fight diseases such as cancer. Immunotherapy may include the use of drugs that stimulate the immune response or the modification of immune cells to attack cancer cells.

Innovation in Patient Care

1. Telemedicine

Telemedicine has transformed the way patients access medical care:

- Remote consultations: Enable patients to receive medical care from the comfort of their home, eliminating geographical barriers. Video consultations can facilitate access to specialists and reduce waiting time for appointments.
- Remote Monitoring: Devices that allow clinicians to monitor chronic conditions such as diabetes and hypertension in real time. Continuous monitoring devices can send data directly to healthcare providers, allowing for immediate adjustments in treatment.
- Digital Health Platforms: Applications and portals that facilitate communication between patients and healthcare providers, access to medical records and appointment management. These platforms can also offer medication reminders and personalised health advice.

2. Wearables and Medical Devices

Wearable devices are playing an increasingly important role in health monitoring:

- Smartwatches: Equipped with sensors that monitor heart rate, physical activity and sleep patterns. These devices can alert users to irregularities in their health and motivate them to stay active.
- Continuous Glucose Monitoring Devices: Allow patients with diabetes to monitor their glucose levels in real time. These devices can send alerts when glucose levels are too high or too low, helping patients to manage their condition more effectively.
- Medical Implants: Devices such as pacemakers and insulin pumps that manage chronic

conditions on an ongoing basis. Advanced implants can be automatically adjusted to optimise patient treatment.

3. Virtual and Augmented Reality

These technologies are finding innovative applications in healthcare:

• Training and Education: Virtual reality simulations for the training of medical students and the continuing education of professionals. These simulations can provide immersive, hands-on learning experiences without risk to patients.

• Therapy and Rehabilitation: Virtual reality programmes used to treat disorders such as PTSD and for physical rehabilitation of injured patients. Virtual reality can create controlled environments for exposure therapy and interactive rehabilitation.

Innovation in Health Management and Logistics

1. Health Information Systems

Health information systems are improving data management and operational efficiency:

• Electronic Health Records (EHR): Facilitate access to and management of patient information, improving care coordination. EHRs allow healthcare providers to access complete and up-to-date medical records, improving clinical decision-making.

• Hospital Management Systems: Software that optimises resource management, staff scheduling and inventory management. These systems can reduce waiting times and improve operational efficiency.

• Big Data Analytics: Using large volumes of data to identify public health trends and improve emergency planning and response. Data analytics can help predict disease outbreaks and optimise the allocation of medical resources.

2. Blockchain in Health

Blockchain technology offers solutions to improve security and transparency in healthcare data management:

• Data Security: Blockchain ensures the integrity and privacy of medical records. By creating an immutable record of transactions, blockchain can prevent fraud and unauthorised access.

• Interoperability: Facilitates the secure exchange of information between different healthcare systems. Enhanced interoperability allows healthcare providers to access accurate and complete patient data, regardless of the system they use.

• Traceability of Medicines: Enables medicines to be tracked from manufacture to patient, reducing the risk of counterfeiting. Blockchain can ensure that medicines are authentic and safe.

3. Logistics and Supply Chain

Technology is optimising the supply chain in the healthcare sector:

• Drones and Robots: Used for the delivery of medicines and medical supplies to hard-to-reach areas. Drones can quickly transport vaccines and medicines to remote regions, while robots can handle logistical tasks within hospitals.

• Inventory Automation: Automated systems for tracking and managing inventories, reducing waste and ensuring the availability of critical supplies. Automation can improve inventory management accuracy and reduce operating costs.

• Demand Forecasting Systems: Algorithms that predict the demand for medicines and medical equipment, improving the efficiency of the supply chain. These systems can anticipate future needs and avoid stock-outs.

Ethical Challenges and Considerations

1. Data Privacy and Security

Handling large amounts of health data poses significant challenges in terms of privacy and security. It is crucial to implement robust measures to protect patient information and ensure its confidentiality. Regulatory frameworks, such as the GDPR in Europe, set standards for the protection of personal data.

2. Access and Inequality

The adoption of new technologies can exacerbate inequalities if equitable access is not ensured. It is vital to develop strategies that ensure that all populations, especially the most vulnerable, can benefit from technological advances. This includes the provision of technological infrastructure in underserved areas and education on the use of new tools.

3. Informed Consent and Autonomy

The use of advanced technologies must be accompanied by sound informed consent practices. Patients must be fully aware of how their data will be used and have the right to opt out of technological programmes if they so wish. This is essential to respect patient autonomy.

4. Sustainability and Cost

While technology can improve the efficiency and quality of health care, it can also entail significant costs. It is essential to assess the economic sustainability of technological innovations and to ensure that the benefits outweigh the costs. Technology adoption must be economically viable and must not compromise accessibility to care.

Conclusion

Innovation and technology are transforming the field of healthcare, offering unprecedented opportunities to improve diagnosis, treatment and care management. However, along with these advances come significant challenges that must be addressed carefully and responsibly from an ethical perspective.The handling of large amounts of health data poses critical challenges in terms of privacy and security. The collection and use of medical data, especially with advanced technologies such as artificial intelligence and big data analytics, require strict security measures to protect patient information. The implementation of robust regulatory frameworks and the adoption of technologies such as blockchain to ensure data integrity and confidentiality are essential. In addition, patients must be informed and give their consent on how their data will be used, thus maintaining their autonomy and trust in the healthcare system.The rapid adoption of new technologies can exacerbate existing inequalities if equitable access is not ensured. It is vital to develop inclusive strategies that ensure that all populations, especially the most vulnerable, can benefit from these advances. This includes the provision of technological infrastructure in underserved areas, education on the use of new tools, and subsidies for technological devices and services. Equity in access to technology is an ethical imperative to avoid creating a digital divide in health. The use of advanced technologies must be accompanied by sound informed consent practices. Patients must be fully aware of how their data will be used and have the right to opt out of technological programmes if they so wish. This is essential to respect patient autonomy and ensure that decisions about their health are made in a free and informed manner. Technologies should be used to empower patients, not to restrict their freedom of choice.While technology can improve the efficiency and quality of health care, it can also entail significant costs. It is essential to assess the economic sustainability of technological innovations and to ensure that the benefits outweigh the costs. Technology adoption must be economically viable and must not compromise accessibility to care. Health systems must strike a balance between investing in new technologies and ensuring that these investments generate tangible benefits for patients. A significant challenge is the interoperability of healthcare technology systems. The ability of different systems and devices to communicate and share information effectively is crucial for coordinated and efficient care. Lack of interoperability can lead to fragmentation of care and duplication of efforts. It is essential to establish standards and protocols that facilitate the integration and secure exchange of data between various technology platforms. Artificial intelligence (AI) and machine learning present unique ethical challenges. AI algorithms must be transparent and fair, avoiding biases that can perpetuate inequities in healthcare. In addition, automated decision-making must be complemented by human clinical judgement, ensuring that critical decisions about patient care are based on a combination of data and empathy. AI should be a tool to enhance the capacity of healthcare professionals, not replace them. The implementation of new health technologies requires a robust governance framework that ensures responsibility and accountability. Technology developers and providers must adhere to strict ethical standards and regulations to protect patients. Health organisations should establish ethics committees and working groups dedicated to assessing the impact of emerging technologies and formulating policies that promote their ethical and responsible use.Finally, it is crucial to consider the social and human impact of health technologies. Technology should be used to improve the quality of life and well-being of patients, not just to optimise the efficiency of the health system. This includes assessing how technologies affect the doctor-patient relationship, the quality of care and the patient experience. Technological advances must be humanised, always keeping the dignity and well-being of individuals at the centre. As we move into an increasingly technological future, it is imperative that healthcare professionals, technology developers, regulators and society at large work together to address these ethical challenges. Collaboration and ongoing dialogue will be essential to ensure that technological innovations benefit all in an equitable and fair manner. Technology has the potential to radically transform healthcare, but only if it is implemented with a firm commitment to ethics and human rights. By harnessing these technologies in an equitable and ethical manner, we can move towards a healthcare system that is not only more efficient and effective, but also more accessible and just for all. In the following chapters, we will explore how these technological advances can be integrated into clinical practice and how health professionals can adapt and contribute to this technological transformation, always with an ethical approach that respects and promotes human dignity and social justice.

CHAPTER 6

HEALTH EDUCATION AND LITERACY FOR ALL INTRODUCTION TO HEALTH LITERACY AND EDUCATION

Education and health literacy are essential components of empowering individuals and communities to manage their well-being. Health literacy refers not only to the ability to read and understand medical information, but also to the ability to apply this knowledge in making informed health decisions. A well-informed population can prevent disease, manage chronic conditions and effectively navigate the health system. This chapter discusses the importance of health education and literacy, the challenges that exist, and strategies to improve these aspects at the individual and collective levels.

Importance of Health Literacy

1. Improving Health Outcomes

High health literacy is correlated with better health outcomes. People who understand health information are more likely to follow medical advice, take their medications correctly and participate in preventive activities. Health education also encourages adherence to treatment and preventive screening, which can lead to earlier diagnosis and more effective disease management.

2. Cost Reduction

Health literacy contributes to cost savings in the health system by reducing the need for emergency interventions and hospitalisations. Well-informed individuals can better manage their chronic conditions and avoid serious complications. In addition, disease prevention through health literacy reduces the financial burden on both individuals and health systems.

3. Promoting Self-Care

Health education encourages self-care, enabling people to take an active role in managing their health. This includes adopting healthy habits, monitoring symptoms and seeking medical care when necessary. Health education also empowers individuals to make informed choices and feel more confident in managing their well-being.

Health Literacy Challenges

1. Complexity of Medical Information

Medical information is often complex and can be difficult to understand for people without specialised training. The use of technical terminology and the lack of clear and accessible educational material are significant barriers. Information overload and variability in the quality of sources can also confuse patients.

2. Socio-economic inequalities

Socio-economic inequalities affect health literacy. People who are less educated, have low incomes or belong to ethnic minorities may have less access to adequate health information and educational resources. These inequalities can perpetuate cycles of poor health and limited access to health care.

3. Access to Information

Access to health information varies significantly between different regions and populations. Rural areas and marginalised communities often lack educational resources and access to the internet, limiting their ability to obtain up-to-date and relevant information. Language and cultural barriers can also hinder access to understandable and useful information.

Strategies to Improve Health Literacy and Education

1. Simplification of Medical Information

It is crucial that medical information is understandable to all levels of literacy. This includes:

• Use of Plain Language: Avoid technical terminology and use simple language. Communication should be direct and easy to understand.

• Visual materials: Use graphics, infographics and videos to explain complex concepts. Visual representations can help clarify information and make it more accessible.

• Translation and Cultural Adaptation: Ensure that information is available in multiple languages and is culturally relevant. Adapting educational materials to the specific needs and contexts of communities can improve understanding and acceptance.

2. Community Education Programmes

Community education programmes are key to improving health literacy:

• Workshops and Seminars: Organise educational events on health issues relevant to the community. These events can be interactive and participatory, encouraging active learning.

• Health promoters: Train community members to act as health promoters, disseminating information and supporting their neighbours. Health promoters can act as effective links between health services and the community.

• Collaboration with Schools and Organisations: Partner with local educational institutions and organisations to integrate health education into their programmes. Schools and community organisations can play a key role in disseminating health information.

3. Use of Technology

Technology can be a powerful tool for improving health education:

• Health Apps: Develop mobile applications that provide health information, medication reminders and educational resources. These apps can offer personalised content that is accessible at any time.

• Telemedicine: Use telemedicine platforms to provide educational consultations and health counselling. Telemedicine can extend the reach of educational services and provide ongoing support.

• Social media: Use social media to disseminate health information and promote healthy habits. Social media campaigns can reach broad and diverse audiences, encouraging engagement and interaction.

4. Promotion of Continuing Education

Health education should be a continuous process throughout life:

• Adult Education Programmes: Offer health education courses and workshops for adults. Continuing education can update people's knowledge and skills in health issues.

• Training for Health Professionals: Ensure that health professionals are trained in effective communication and health education. Professionals should be prepared to explain medical concepts in a clear and understandable manner.

• Awareness Campaigns: Conduct regular campaigns to raise awareness of the importance of health literacy. Campaigns can use a variety of media to disseminate key messages and motivate learning.

Examples of Successful Initiatives

1. Health Literacy Project in the United States

The Health Literacy Project is an initiative designed to improve health literacy in low-income communities in the United States. This project provides a variety of educational resources and tools to help people better understand and manage their health. Health Literacy Project activities include:

• Educational Workshops: Community workshops are organised where basic health skills are taught, such as how to read medicine labels, interpret medical test results and understand medical instructions. These workshops are interactive and designed to be accessible to people with different literacy levels.

• Educational Materials: The project develops and distributes clear and easy-to-understand educational materials, including educational booklets, guides and videos. These materials are available in multiple languages and are culturally adapted to be relevant to the communities they serve.

• Personalised Support: Through community health advisors, the project offers individualised support to help people navigate the health system, manage their chronic conditions and make informed decisions about their health. Counsellors work directly with individuals to provide guidance and address questions.

• Training Programmes: The Health Literacy Project also offers training programmes for health professionals, teaching them how to communicate medical information effectively and how to better support patients with low health literacy.

The impact of the Health Literacy Project has been significant, demonstrating improvements in the understanding and management of health among the populations. vulnerable people, reducing hospitalisation rates and improving adherence to medical treatment.

2. Health Promoters in Latin America

In many Latin American countries, health promoters play a key role in community education and in improving health literacy. These promoters are usually community members who have received specific training in health issues and act as liaisons between the community and the health system. Some salient characteristics and activities of health promoters include:

• Community training: Health promoters receive training in various areas of health, including disease prevention, management of chronic conditions, reproductive health and first aid. This training enables them to effectively educate and assist their neighbours.

• Home visits: Promotores make visits to people's homes to provide information and personalised support. These visits allow for a more individualised approach and can address the specific needs of each family.

• Workshops and Talks: Organise and facilitate workshops and talks on health topics relevant to the community, promoting healthy practices and disease prevention. These events also provide a space for community members to ask questions and receive trusted answers.

• Public Health Campaigns: Promotores participate in public health campaigns, distributing educational materials and helping to organise community events such as vaccination days, health fairs and disease screening programmes.

The health promoter model has proven to be extremely effective in improving health literacy and promoting health practices.

The project aims to improve health outcomes in rural and urban communities in Latin America by reducing gaps in access to information and improving health outcomes.

3. Doctoralia" application in Spain

Doctoralia is a digital platform that has revolutionised access to health information in Spain and other countries. The application allows users to search for information on diseases, treatments and health professionals, offering a space for interaction between patients and doctors. Some of Doctoralia's outstanding features include:

• Health Professional Search: Users can search and find doctors and specialists in various health areas, view their profiles, read reviews from other patients and make appointments online. This facilitates access to trusted professionals and allows patients to make informed decisions about their healthcare.

• Health Information: Doctoralia provides a vast database of information on symptoms, diseases and treatments, written in clear and accessible language. This information is reviewed by medical professionals, ensuring accuracy and relevance.

• Patient-Physician Interaction: The platform allows patients to ask questions to doctors and receive answers online. This function is particularly useful for clarifying doubts and obtaining medical advice without the need to travel.

• Appointment Management: Doctoralia facilitates the management of medical appointments, allowing users to schedule, modify or cancel appointments easily and quickly. It also sends automatic reminders, helping patients to keep their appointments and follow their treatment plans.

Doctoralia has significantly improved access to quality health information and facilitated communication between patients and healthcare professionals. health, contributing to increased health literacy and informed decision-making.

Performance of Health Professionals

1. Effective Communication

Health professionals must develop effective communication skills to convey medical information in a clear and understandable manner. This includes:

• Active Listening: Paying attention to patients' concerns and questions. Active listening helps to build trust and better understand patients' needs.

• Explain clearly: Use simple language and ensure that patients understand the information provided. Practitioners should avoid using medical jargon and be clear in their explanations.

• Confirm Understanding: Ask patients to repeat the information back to ensure that they have understood correctly. The "teach-back" technique is useful to verify understanding.

2. Education and Counselling

Health professionals should play an active role in educating their patients:

• Educational sessions: Offer educational sessions during consultations to explain diagnosis, treatment and preventive measures. Educational sessions may include practical demonstrations and supporting materials.

• Educational materials: Provide handouts, videos and other educational materials for patients to review at home. Materials should be clear, concise and easy to understand.

• Ongoing support: Provide follow-up and ongoing support to help patients implement and maintain healthy habits. Ongoing support may include follow-up calls, text messages and appointment reminders.

Conclusion

Education and health literacy are fundamental to improving the health and wellbeing of individuals and communities. By addressing existing barriers and employing effective strategies, we can empower individuals to make informed decisions about their health and adopt self-care practices. From an ethical perspective, it is essential to ensure that all people, regardless of their socio-economic or cultural background, have access to the information and resources they need to manage their health effectively. It is a mandatory duty of health professionals to take the lead in designing and implementing health education programmes. These programmes should take advantage of all available means, including community workshops, educational materials, digital technology and social media, to reach diverse populations and ensure that information is delivered effectively. The responsibility of health professionals is not limited to clinical care; it also includes the mission to educate and guide patients and communities towards better understanding and management of their health. Healthcare professionals play a crucial role in this process, and their commitment to education and effective communication can make a significant difference to the lives of their patients. By creating and disseminating clear and accessible educational materials, and through ongoing training in communication skills, professionals can ensure that their patients understand and can act on the health information they receive. Health literacy not only improves individual outcomes, but also strengthens communities and contributes to health equity. A well-informed population is better equipped to prevent disease, manage chronic conditions and actively participate in their care. In addition, health literacy promotes social justice by ensuring that everyone, regardless of socio-economic status, has an equal opportunity to reach their full health potential.

CHAPTER 7

INTERSECTORAL COLLABORATION FOR HEALTH PROMOTION INTRODUCTION TO INTERSECTORAL COLLABORATION

Health promotion is a collective effort that transcends the boundaries of the health sector. Intersectoral collaboration involves cooperation across sectors, such as education, housing, transport and the environment, to address the social determinants of health and create environments that support wellbeing. This approach recognises that health is influenced by a wide range of factors and that joint action can have a significant impact on improving health outcomes.

Importance of Intersectoral Collaboration

1. Addressing the Social Determinants of Health

The social determinants of health, such as education, employment, housing and the physical environment, have a profound impact on people's health. Cross-sectoral collaboration enables these determinants to be addressed in a comprehensive manner, promoting an environment that supports health and well-being. By working together, sectors can identify and address the underlying causes of health disparities, such as poverty, inequality and limited access to essential resources.

2. Resource Optimisation

Collaboration between different sectors allows for a more efficient use of available resources. By combining efforts and sharing knowledge, more effective and sustainable solutions can be developed. Optimising resources not only reduces costs, but also maximises the impact of interventions, ensuring that benefits reach the populations that need them most.

3. Innovation and Creativity

Interaction between diverse sectors fosters innovation and creativity in the development of health interventions. The unique perspectives of each sector can contribute to innovative and more effective solutions. Diversity of ideas and approaches can lead to the creation of more comprehensive programmes tailored to the specific needs of the community.

Models and Strategies for Intersectoral Collaboration

1. Collaborative Governance Models

Collaborative governance models provide a structure for cross-sectoral cooperation. These models include:

- Intersectoral Committees: Working groups made up of representatives from different sectors that meet regularly to plan and coordinate actions. These committees can develop integrated strategies and oversee their implementation.

• Public-Private Partnerships: Collaborations between the public sector and private companies to address specific health challenges. These partnerships can mobilise additional resources and leverage private sector expertise.

• Community Networks: Coalitions of community organisations working together to promote health in their community. Community networks can foster local participation and ensure that interventions are culturally relevant.

2. Community-Based Approaches

Community-based approaches involve community members in the design and implementation of health interventions. This includes:

• Community Participation: Involve residents in identifying health problems and deciding on solutions. Active community participation ensures that interventions are accepted and sustainable.

• Community Empowerment: Strengthening community capacities to lead and sustain health initiatives. Empowerment builds community self-efficacy and resilience.

3. Policy Integration

Policy integration involves coordinating policies across sectors to promote health. Strategies include:

• Health in All Policies (HiAP): An approach that incorporates health considerations into all policy areas, from urban planning to education to transport. This approach ensures that policies in all sectors contribute to improving public health.

• Health Impact Assessment (HIA): A tool that assesses the potential health consequences of a policy, plan or project in any sector, with the aim of improving health outcomes. HIA can identify opportunities to mitigate negative impacts and maximise health benefits.

Examples of Intersectoral Collaboration

1. Healthy Schools Programmes

Schools can be a crucial setting for health promotion. Healthy schools programmes involve collaboration between the education sector and the health sector to:

• Health Education: Include health issues in the school curriculum. This can range from nutrition and physical activity to mental health and disease prevention.

• Healthy School Environments: Improve nutrition and promote physical activity in schools. This may include implementing healthy lunch programmes and creating spaces for exercise and active play.

• School Health Services: Provide mental and physical health services within schools. Services may include school nurses, counsellors and health screening programmes.

2. Healthy Housing Projects

The quality of housing has a significant impact on health. Healthy housing projects, which involve collaboration between the housing sector and the health sector, can:

• Improve Indoor Air Quality: Reduce pollutants and improve ventilation. This may involve removing mould and installing adequate ventilation systems.

• Ensure Housing Safety: Eliminate safety hazards and improve accessibility. This may include repairing dangerous structures and installing ramps and grab bars.

• Promote Safe and Healthy Environments: Create green spaces and recreational areas. Green spaces not only improve physical health, but also mental well-being.

3. Transport and Health

The transport sector also plays an important role in public health. Healthy transport initiatives can include:

• Active Transport Promotion: Promote cycling and walking by creating appropriate infrastructure. This may include the construction of bicycle lanes and the improvement of pavements.

• Air Pollution Reduction: Implement policies to reduce vehicle emissions and promote the use of public transport. This may involve the development of efficient and accessible public transport systems.

• Road Safety: Implement measures to reduce traffic accidents and improve road safety. Measures may include the installation of traffic lights, the creation of low speed zones and road safety education.

Benefits of Cross-Sectoral Collaboration

1. Improving Population Health

Intersectoral interventions can more effectively address the social determinants of health, improving health outcomes at the population level. By working together, sectors can create environments that promote health and prevent disease.

2. Reducing Health Inequities

Intersectoral collaboration can help reduce health inequities by ensuring that resources and interventions reach the most vulnerable and disadvantaged populations. Health equity is strengthened when all sectors contribute to removing barriers to accessing quality care.

3. Strengthening Social Cohesion

Working together across sectors and community participation can strengthen social cohesion and foster a sense of shared ownership and responsibility. Intersectoral collaboration not only improves health, but also builds more cohesive and resilient communities.

Challenges and Barriers to Intersectoral Collaboration

1. Differences in Objectives and Priorities

Each sector has its own objectives and priorities, which can make alignment and effective collaboration difficult. It is essential to find common ground and work towards shared goals.

2. Lack of Communication and Coordination

Lack of communication and coordination between sectors can result in fragmented efforts and duplication of resources. Establishing clear communication channels and coordination mechanisms can mitigate these problems.

3. Structural and Cultural Barriers

Structural and cultural differences between sectors can be significant barriers to collaboration. Strategies need to be developed to overcome these differences and foster a collaborative environment.

Strategies for Overcoming Barriers

1. Establishing Common Objectives

Defining common objectives that benefit all sectors involved can help align priorities and foster collaboration. Shared objectives should be clear, achievable and measurable.

2. Improving Communication and Coordination

Developing clear and efficient communication channels and establishing coordination mechanisms can improve collaboration between sectors. Regular meetings and communication platforms can facilitate information exchange and joint decision-making.

3. Training and Awareness Raising

Training actors from different sectors on the importance of cross-sectoral collaboration and raising awareness of the benefits of working together can help overcome cultural and structural barriers. Ongoing training and team-building activities can strengthen collaboration.

Conclusion

Intersectoral collaboration is essential for effective health promotion. By pooling efforts and resources across sectors, we can comprehensively address the social determinants of health and create environments that support wellbeing. Health professionals have a crucial role in leading and supporting these initiatives, ensuring that policies and programmes are developed and implemented effectively and equitably.Specifically, health professionals should take leadership roles in forming and coordinating intersectoral committees and partnerships, convening meetings and facilitating dialogues between representatives from different sectors to discuss strategies and coordinate efforts. In addition, they should collaborate with other sectors to create integrated action plans that address the social determinants of health, delegate clear tasks and responsibilities to the different actors involved, and ensure that each sector contributes meaningfully.Evaluation and monitoring of cross-sectoral interventions are key tasks for health professionals. They should develop performance indicators to measure the impact of interventions, conduct periodic evaluations to monitor progress and make necessary adjustments to programmes, and share findings with all stakeholders, using the data to improve future interventions.Leading the education and training of other sectors on health issues is another key aspect. Health professionals should develop training programmes for actors in other sectors to understand the social determinants of health and how their actions can influence the well-being of the community. They should also promote health literacy, ensuring that health information is accessible and understandable to all sectors involved, and raise awareness of the importance of intersectoral collaboration and the benefits of working together to improve public health. In terms of implementing intersectoral policies and programmes, health professionals should work to integrate health policies across all areas of government, ensuring that decisions in sectors such as transport, education and housing take into account their impact on health. They must establish clear and efficient communication mechanisms across sectors to ensure smooth implementation of programmes and provide technical advice and support to ensure that interventions are based on the best available evidence and tailored to the specific needs of the community.Encouraging active community participation in health initiatives is also an important responsibility. Health professionals must ensure that community members have a say in the planning and implementation of health interventions, provide tools and resources for the community to lead and sustain health initiatives over the long term, and keep the community informed about the progress and outcomes of interventions, with transparent accountability. Although challenges and barriers exist, the strategies described in this chapter can help overcome them and foster successful cooperation. Intersectoral collaboration not only improves health outcomes, but also strengthens social cohesion and fosters a sense of ownership and shared responsibility.

CHAPTER 8

SUSTAINABILITY AND RESILIENCE IN GLOBAL HEALTH AN INTRODUCTION TO SUSTAINABILITY AND RESILIENCE IN HEALTH

Sustainability and resilience are fundamental concepts in the field of global health. Sustainability in health refers to the ability of health systems to maintain and improve standards of care over time without compromising the ability of future generations to meet their own health needs. Resilience, on the other hand, refers to the ability of health systems to adapt and respond effectively to crises, disasters and environmental change. In this chapter, we will explore the importance of these concepts, current challenges, and strategies to foster sustainability and resilience in global health.

Importance of Sustainability in Health

1. Limited Resources

Resources for health care are limited and must be managed efficiently to ensure that they are available for the long term. Sustainability ensures that health systems can operate continuously without depleting natural, economic and human resources.

2. Climate Change and Health

Climate change has a significant impact on global health, affecting the availability of clean water, food security and the spread of disease. Sustainability in health includes strategies to mitigate these impacts and adapt to new environmental realities.

3. Intergenerational Equity

Sustainability also involves considering the well-being of future generations. A sustainable approach to health ensures that today's decisions do not compromise the ability of future generations to enjoy good health.

Importance of Resilience in Health

1. Crisis and Disaster Response

Resilient health systems can respond effectively to crises and disasters, minimising the impact on the population. This includes preparedness for pandemics, natural disasters and conflict.

2. Adaptability

Resilience enables health systems to adapt to rapid change and meet emerging challenges, such as new diseases, demographic shifts and changes in resource availability.

3. Continuity of Care

Resilient health systems ensure continuity of care even in adverse situations, protecting the most vulnerable populations and maintaining essential services.

Challenges to Sustainability and Resilience in Global Health

1. Inadequate funding

Inadequate financing and lack of investment in robust health infrastructure are major obstacles to sustainability and resilience. Without adequate financial resources, it is difficult to maintain quality health services and respond to emergencies.

2. Health Inequalities

Health inequalities, both within and between countries, make it difficult to implement sustainable and resilient strategies. Vulnerable populations often lack access to adequate health services and are most affected by crises and disasters.

3. Climate Change

Climate change presents significant challenges to global health, exacerbating existing diseases and facilitating the emergence of new ones. Health systems must adapt rapidly to these changes to protect populations.

4. Governance and Policy

Lack of effective governance and integrated health policies can limit the ability of health systems to be sustainable and resilient. Coordination and planning at local, national and international levels are essential.

Strategies to Promote Health Sustainability

1. Energy Efficiency and Emission Reduction

Implementing energy efficiency practices in healthcare facilities and reducing carbon emissions are crucial steps towards sustainability. This includes the use of renewable energy sources such as solar and wind, the design and construction of sustainable healthcare facilities that minimise environmental impact, and the implementation of effective waste management practices to reduce environmental impact.

2. Resource Conservation

Sustainable management of resources such as water and medical supplies is essential. Strategies include the rational use of water by implementing water saving and recycling systems in healthcare facilities, and the optimisation of medical materials for efficient use and waste reduction.

3. Health Promotion and Prevention

Investing in health promotion and disease prevention can reduce the burden on health systems and improve long-term sustainability. This includes expanding vaccination coverage to prevent infectious diseases and the promotion of healthy lifestyles through health education programmes.

Strategies to Strengthen Resilience in Health

1. Emergency Preparedness

Developing and maintaining emergency preparedness plans is essential for resilience. This includes establishing contingency plans with clear protocols for responding to different types of crises, and training health staff through regular drills to ensure preparedness.

2. Resilient Infrastructure

Developing health infrastructures that can withstand disasters and continue to operate in adverse conditions is crucial. This includes designing health facilities that are resistant to natural disasters such as earthquakes and floods, and implementing back-up systems for electricity, water and communications.

3. International Collaboration

Collaboration at the international level is crucial to address global challenges and strengthen resilience. This includes sharing information and best practices between countries and international organisations, and establishing cooperative arrangements to provide mutual assistance in times of crisis.

Examples of Sustainability and Resilience in Health

1. Costa Rican Health System

Costa Rica is recognised for its sustainable and resilient health system. The country has achieved universal health coverage through the Caja Costarricense de Seguro Social (CCSS), which finances and administers most of the country's health services. Investment in renewable energy has been a key pillar of Costa Rica's sustainability. Approximately 99% of the country's electricity comes from renewable sources such as hydro, geothermal, wind and solar. This energy transition has not only reduced carbon emissions, but also improved air quality and, consequently, public health.

In addition, Costa Rica has implemented effective public health policies that promote prevention and self-care. Universal vaccination programmes and health education campaigns have significantly reduced the incidence of infectious and chronic diseases. The health infrastructure has also been designed to be resilient, with hospitals and health centres built to withstand earthquakes and other natural disasters. Costa Rica has demonstrated how investment in sustainable infrastructure and the promotion of public health policies can improve the health and resilience of the health system.

2. Emergency Preparedness in Japan

Japan has developed one of the most advanced disaster preparedness systems in the world, based on its experience with earthquakes, tsunamis and other natural disasters. Health infrastructures in Japan are designed to withstand major earthquakes and tsunamis, thanks to strict construction standards and the use of advanced engineering technologies. Hospitals and health centres are equipped with emergency systems and contingency plans to ensure that they can continue to operate during and after a disaster.

Japan conducts regular national and local drills to prepare citizens and health professionals for various emergencies. These drills include evacuation drills, first aid training and simulation of mass disaster response. In addition, the Japanese government has established an early warning system that uses advanced technology to detect earthquakes and tsunamis, enabling a rapid and effective response. Japan's focus on emergency preparedness and the resilient infrastructure serves as a model for other countries seeking to improve their disaster response capacity.

3. Health Programmes in Rwanda

Rwanda has implemented innovative programmes to strengthen its health system and improve resilience, especially in rural areas. One of the pillars of these efforts has been the training of community health workers. These workers are members of local communities who are specifically trained to provide primary care, health education and chronic disease management support. Their presence in communities has significantly improved access to health services and enabled a faster and more effective response to health emergencies.

Rwanda has also embraced the use of mobile technologies to improve healthcare. The country's health system uses mobile applications for patient tracking, medical supply management and communication between health professionals. These technologies have facilitated the delivery of health services in remote areas and improved the efficiency of the health system. In addition, Rwanda has implemented a community health insurance programme that has increased health coverage and reduced financial barriers to accessing health care. The combination of training community health workers, the use of mobile technologies and the implementation of health insurance has strengthened the resilience of Rwanda's health system and provided more equitable access to health services. These efforts have resulted in significant improvements in health indicators, such as reduced maternal and infant mortality and increased life expectancy.

Conclusion

Sustainability and resilience are essential to ensure long-term health and well-being in an ever-changing world. By implementing effective strategies and addressing current challenges, health systems can become more robust and able to respond to emergencies, while protecting the well-being of future generations. Health professionals have a crucial role in this process, leading and supporting initiatives to improve sustainability and resilience. This includes planning and coordinating efforts, implementing integrated health policies, promoting sustainable practices and preparing for emergencies.Furthermore, it is imperative that governments show strong political will to address these challenges. The adoption of sustainable and resilient health policies requires the commitment of government leaders to adequately finance health systems, invest in robust infrastructure and promote health equity. Governments must establish regulatory frameworks that incentivise sustainability and resilience, and foster international collaboration to address shared global challenges. Political will is crucial to ensure that policies and programmes are implemented effectively and equitably, benefiting all populations, especially the most vulnerable. Intersectoral collaboration and international cooperation are also key components of building sustainable and resilient health systems. By working together and harnessing technological innovations, we can move towards a global health system that is sustainable, resilient and equitable for all.

CHAPTER 9

ETHICS AND HUMAN RIGHTS IN HEALTHCARE INTRODUCTION TO ETHICS AND HUMAN RIGHTS IN HEALTHCARE

Ethics and human rights are fundamental pillars of health care. Health ethics encompasses the principles and values that guide the conduct of health professionals, while human rights ensure that all people are treated with dignity and equity in access to health services. In this chapter, we will explore key ethical principles, the importance of human rights in health, challenges and strategies for integrating these concepts into daily practice.

Ethical Principles in Health Care

1. Autonomy

The principle of autonomy recognises the right of patients to make informed decisions about their own health. This includes:

• Informed Consent: Patients should receive all necessary information about their diagnosis, treatment options and potential risks in order to make informed decisions. Health professionals have a responsibility to provide this information in a clear and understandable manner.

• Respect for Patient Decisions: Health professionals should respect patients' decisions, even if they do not agree with them, as long as patients are fully informed and competent to make such decisions. This also implies respecting patients' cultural and personal preferences.

2. Charity

Beneficence refers to the obligation of health professionals to act in the best interests of patients. This includes:

• Providing the Best Possible Care: Professionals should strive to provide the most effective and safe care, making optimal use of available resources.

• Risk-Benefit Assessment: Treatments and procedures must be carefully evaluated to ensure that the benefits outweigh the risks. This involves constant updating and continuing education on medical and therapeutic advances.

3. Non-Maleficence

The principle of non-maleficence states that health professionals should avoid causing harm to patients. This includes:

• Risk Minimisation: Practitioners should take all necessary precautions to avoid complications and adverse effects, including adherence to clinical protocols and guidelines.

• Evidence-Based Practice: Use treatments and procedures based on the best available scientific evidence to minimise the risk of harm. Informed, evidence-based decision making is fundamental to this principle.

4. Justice

Justice in health refers to the equitable distribution of resources and access to care. This includes:

• Equity in Access to Care: Ensuring that all patients have access to quality health services, regardless of socio-economic background, race, gender or sexual orientation.

• Fair Resource Allocation: Health resources must be allocated fairly and equitably, prioritising the needs of the most vulnerable. This implies public health policies that address inequalities and promote equity.

Human Rights in Health

1. Right to Health

The right to health is a fundamental human right recognised by numerous international instruments, including the Universal Declaration of Human Rights and the International Covenant on Economic, Social and Cultural Rights. This right entails:

• Access to Health Services: All people should have access to affordable, accessible and quality health services. This includes the availability of essential medicines and appropriate treatment.

• Social Determinants of Health: The right to health also includes access to the social determinants of health, such as safe drinking water, adequate food, housing and a healthy environment. Governments must implement policies that address these determinants to improve public health.

2. Non-discrimination

The principle of non-discrimination is essential to ensure equal access to health services. This includes:

• Equal Treatment: All patients must be treated with equality and respect, without discrimination on the basis of race, gender, sexual orientation, disability, religion or socio-economic status.

• Inclusive Access: Health systems must be designed to be inclusive and accessible to all people, including those with disabilities and other special needs. This involves removing physical and cultural barriers that impede access to care.

3. Confidentiality and Privacy

Confidentiality and privacy are fundamental rights of patients. This includes:

• Protection of Medical Information: Health professionals must ensure that patients' medical information is kept confidential and is only shared with the patient's consent.

• Privacy in Care: Ensure that patients have privacy during medical care, including consultations and procedures. Protecting privacy strengthens patient trust in the health care system.

Challenges in Integrating Ethics and Human Rights

1. Limited Resources

Resource scarcity can make it difficult to implement ethical principles and human rights, especially in environments with economic constraints and lack of infrastructure. Prioritising resources and making difficult decisions are constant challenges.

2. Social and Economic Inequalities

Social and economic inequalities can prevent certain groups from accessing quality health services, violating the principle of justice and the right to health. It is essential to address these inequalities through inclusive and equitable policies.

3. Cultural and Religious Conflicts

Cultural and religious differences may lead to conflicts in the application of ethical principles, especially with regard to patient autonomy and informed decision-making. Cultural awareness and respect for patients' beliefs are essential to resolve these conflicts.

4. Lack of Education and Training

The lack of education and training in ethics and human rights among health professionals can lead to the violation of these principles andrights, affecting the quality of care. It is crucial to invest in the continuous training of health professionals on these issues.

Strategies for Promoting Ethics and Human Rights

1. Education and Training

Implement ethics and human rights education and training programmes for all health professionals. This includes:

• Continuing Education: Offer regular courses and workshops on ethics and human rights issues.

• Incorporation in curricula: Include ethics and human rights modules in training programmes for health professionals. Ethics training should be a central component of medical and health education.

2. Policies and Protocols

Develop and implement clear policies and protocols that promote ethics and human rights in health care. This includes:

- Ethical Guidelines: Create ethical guidelines to guide the conduct of health professionals.

- Whistleblowing Procedures: Establish clear procedures for the reporting and resolution of ethical and human rights violations. Accessible and protected reporting channels are essential to maintaining the integrity of the health system.

3. Community Involvement

Engage the community in the promotion and defence of ethics and human rights in health. This includes:

- Community Consultations: Conduct regular consultations with the community to identify needs and concerns.
- Human Rights Advocates: Train community members to act as advocates for human rights in health. Community participation strengthens the legitimacy and effectiveness of health policies.

4. Monitoring and Evaluation

Establish monitoring and evaluation systems to ensure compliance with ethical principles and human rights. This includes:

- Regular Audits: Conduct periodic audits to assess adherence to ethical policies and protocols.

- Impact Evaluations: Assessing the impact of interventions and policies on the promotion of ethics and human rights. Ongoing evaluation is crucial to improve health practices and policies.

Examples of Application of Ethics and Human Rights in Health

1. Geneva Declaration

The Declaration of Geneva, adopted by the World Medical Association, is an ethical commitment for health professionals that emphasises the importance of human rights and ethics in medical practice. This declaration establishes fundamental principles that guide the ethical conduct of physicians throughout the world.

2. Non-Discrimination Initiatives in South Africa

South Africa has implemented initiatives to combat discrimination in the health system by ensuring equitable access to health services for all populations, especially those affected by HIV/AIDS. These initiatives include sensitisation programmes, staff training and inclusion policies.

3. Informed Consent Programmes in Canada

Canada has developed comprehensive informed consent programmes that ensure that patients receive all the information they need to make autonomous decisions about their medical care. These programmes include training health professionals in communication skills and creating accessible information materials for patients.

Conclusion

The integration of ethics and human rights in health care is essential to ensure equitable, respectful and quality care. These principles are not only moral foundations, but also essential to building just and sustainable health systems. Health care must be guided by a deep respect for human dignity, equity and social justice, ensuring that all individuals, regardless of socio-economic background, gender, race or status, have access to quality health services. Continuing education and training in ethics and human rights is crucial for all health professionals. Training should include not only the theoretical foundations, but also the practical application of these principles in everyday situations. Health professionals must be prepared to confront ethical dilemmas with competence and sensitivity, and to defend the rights of their patients with integrity and courage.The development of clear policies and protocols that promote ethics and human rights is essential. These policies should be designed to protect patients and guide health professionals in making ethical decisions. Accessible and protected complaints procedures are essential to ensure that any violation of patients' rights can be reported and effectively addressed. Community participation in the promotion and defence of ethics and human rights in health is equally vital. Regular community consultations identify the needs and concerns of the population, ensuring that health policies and programmes are relevant to the needs of the population. and effective. Training of human rights defenders within the community strengthens society's capacity to demand and maintain high standards of care.Ongoing monitoring and evaluation is necessary to ensure compliance with ethical principles and human rights. Regular audits and impact assessments allow for identifying areas for improvement and adjusting policies and practices to maintain quality of care. These processes also provide transparency and accountability, strengthening public confidence in the health system.International examples, such as the Geneva Declaration, non-discrimination initiatives in South Africa and informed consent programmes in Canada, highlight how different countries and organisations have adopted and promoted ethical and human rights principles in their health systems. These examples serve as role models and offer valuable lessons on how to integrate these principles effectively. In addition, it is essential that governments show strong political will to support these initiatives. Adopting health policies that respect and promote human rights requires a genuine commitment from political leaders to adequately finance health systems, invest in robust infrastructure and promote equity in health. Political will is crucial to ensure that policies and programmes are implemented effectively and equitably, benefiting all populations, especially the most vulnerable. Promoting ethics and human rights in health not only improves individual health outcomes, but also strengthens communities and contributes to social justice. A human rights approach ensures that everyone has the opportunity to reach their full health potential, which in turn strengthens social cohesion and fosters a sense of shared ownership and responsibility.

CHAPTER 10

GLOBAL ACTION AND SOLIDARITY IN PUBLIC HEALTH INTRODUCTION TO GLOBAL ACTION AND SOLIDARITY IN HEALTH

Health is a global issue that transcends borders and requires a coordinated and supportive international response. Global action in public health involves collaboration between countries, international organisations, non-governmental entities and the private sector to address the world's most pressing health challenges. Solidarity in public health is the principle underlying this collaboration, recognising that the health and well-being of all people are interconnected. In this chapter, we explore the importance of global action and solidarity in public health, current challenges and strategies to promote effective and equitable collaboration.

Importance of Global Health Action

1. Interconnectedness of Health Problems

Diseases do not respect borders. Pandemics, such as COVID-19, and other public health crises have shown how health problems in one country can affect the rest of the world. Global action is essential to control the spread of infectious diseases and to address health problems that have global implications. International cooperation can facilitate the implementation of control and prevention measures, and ensure a rapid and coordinated response to health emergencies.

2. Resource and Knowledge Sharing

Global action enables the sharing of resources and knowledge, facilitating access to advanced medical technologies, essential medicines and best practices. International collaboration can accelerate research and development of treatments and vaccines, benefiting humanity as a whole. In addition, technology transfer and local capacity building are critical to strengthening health systems in low- and middle-income countries.

3. Promoting Equity in Health

Global action and solidarity in public health promotes equity, ensuring that low- and middle-income countries have access to the resources needed to improve the health of their populations. This equitable approach is crucial to reducing global health inequities. Equity in health is not only a matter of social justice, but also of efficiency, as more equitable health systems tend to be more resilient and effective.

Principles of Solidarity in Public Health

1. Social Justice

Social justice is a fundamental principle of public health solidarity. It implies a commitment to ensuring that all people, regardless of their background, have equal access to health services and the social determinants of health. Social justice also requires addressing health disparities and implementing policies that promote equity and inclusion.

2. Shared Responsibility

Shared responsibility is essential for global action on health. Countries and international organisations must work together, taking responsibility and committing to support those who lack the resources to address their health challenges. Shared responsibility also implies a commitment to transparency and accountability in the implementation of health programmes.

3. Respect and Cooperation

Solidarity in public health is based on mutual respect and cooperation. This means valuing the perspectives and contributions of all actors, and working together in an inclusive and collaborative manner. International cooperation should be guided by principles of equity and fairness, ensuring that that all voices are heard and that decisions are taken in a participatory and consensual manner.

Challenges for Global Action and Health Solidarity

1. Economic and Social Inequalities

Economic and social inequalities between countries can hinder collaboration and equitable access to health resources. Low- and middle-income countries often lack the infrastructure and financial resources needed to implement effective health programmes. It is essential that global action efforts include financing mechanisms that address these inequities and promote economic and social justice.

2. Conflicts and Disasters

Armed conflicts and natural disasters can destabilise health systems and hamper the delivery of health services. Global action must include strategies to support countries in crisis and rebuild their health systems. Humanitarian assistance and cooperation in reconstruction are crucial components of a supportive and effective response.

3. Political and Cultural Barriers

Political and cultural differences can complicate international cooperation. Mistrust, protectionist policies and cultural barriers can impede the implementation of coordinated and effective health programmes. It is crucial to develop approaches that respect cultural diversities and promote dialogue and collaboration between different actors and contexts.

Strategies to Promote Global Action and Health Solidarity

1. Strengthening International Institutions

International institutions, such as the World Health Organisation (WHO), play a crucial role in coordinating global action on health. It is essential to strengthen these institutions, ensuring that they have the resources and mandate to lead global health efforts. This includes adequate funding, inclusive governance and the capacity for rapid and effective response.

2. Public-Private Partnerships

Public-private partnerships can mobilise additional resources and leverage innovation to address health challenges. These partnerships should be equitable and transparent, with a focus on the well-being of the most vulnerable populations. Collaboration with the private sector can include the development and distribution of medicines and health technologies, as well as the implementation of community health programmes.

3. Promoting Research and Development

Investment in research and development (R&D) is essential to address global health challenges. Countries and organisations must collaborate to fund and support R&D, sharing knowledge and technologies for common benefit. Collaborative research can accelerate the development of new therapies and vaccines, and improve our understanding of diseases and their determinants.

4. Training and Education

Training health professionals and educating communities is critical to the sustainability of health programmes. Comprehensive action must include efforts to strengthen local capacity and empower communities through education and training. Continuous training of health professionals and community health education are key to building resilient and sustainable health systems.

Examples of Global Action and Health Solidarity

1. COVAX Initiative

The COVAX initiative is a global effort to ensure equitable access to COVID-19 vaccines. Led by the World Health Organization (WHO), Gavi, the Vaccine Alliance, and the Coalition for Epidemic Preparedness Innovations (CEPI), COVAX has worked tirelessly to deliver vaccines to low- and middle-income countries. Its goal is to ensure that all countries have access to vaccines, regardless of their economic capacity.

Since its launch, COVAX has distributed millions of doses of vaccines in more than 190 countries. The initiative has faced logistical challenges, including supply chain issues and the need for adequate infrastructure for vaccine storage and transport, especially in resource-constrained regions. Despite these challenges, COVAX has been instrumental in ensuring that the most vulnerable countries are not excluded from access to vaccines, demonstrating the importance of global solidarity in responding to pandemics.

The cooperation of multiple actors, including governments, international organisations and the private sector, has enabled COVAX to mobilise resources and ensure equitable distribution of vaccines. In addition, COVAX has promoted technology transfer and local capacity building, supporting countries to develop their own vaccination infrastructures.

2. Malaria Control Programme

The malaria control programme is an outstanding example of global action and solidarity. Collaboration between WHO, national governments, non-governmental organisations (NGOs) and the private sector has significantly reduced the incidence of malaria in many parts of the world. Malaria, which mainly affects tropical countries, is a major cause of death in many parts of the world. The disease has been one of the main causes of infant mortality in these countries.

Coordinated efforts include the distribution of insecticide-treated mosquito nets, which are essential to prevent bites from malaria-transmitting mosquitoes. In addition, access to effective treatments such as artemisinin-based combination therapy (ACT), the first-line treatment for malaria, has been ensured. Prevention and community education campaigns have been crucial to inform communities about prevention measures and the importance of timely treatment.

In areas of high transmission, epidemiological surveillance and investigation have played a vital role in identifying and responding to outbreaks. Funding and technical support from international donors and organisations such as the Global Fund to Fight AIDS, Tuberculosis and Malaria have been essential to sustain these efforts. As a result, many countries have seen a dramatic decline in the incidence of malaria, saving millions of lives and improving the health and well-being of affected populations.

3. Global Alliance for Vaccines and Immunisation (Gavi)

Gavi is a public-private partnership working to increase access to immunisation in low-income countries. Since its inception in 2000, Gavi has immunised hundreds of millions of children against preventable diseases such as measles, polio and rotavirus, preventing disease and improving global health.

Through its focus on equity and innovation, Gavi has strengthened health systems and contributed to reducing child mortality and improving quality of life. The partnership has facilitated the introduction of new vaccines into national immunisation programmes, ensuring that advances in science and technology benefit everyone, regardless of where they were born.

Gavi has also promoted long-term sustainability through co-financing with recipient countries, promoting national ownership and the integration of vaccines into public health systems. In addition, the partnership has supported cold chain infrastructure and health worker training, ensuring that vaccines are properly stored and administered.

Collaboration with industry partners has enabled Gavi to negotiate lower prices for vaccines, making them more affordable for developing countries. This strategy has been instrumental in increasing immunisation coverage and protecting more children against preventable diseases.

The Role of Health Professionals in Global Action

1. Advocacy and Leadership

Health professionals have a crucial role as advocates and leaders in global health action. They can influence policy, engage in international collaborative efforts and advocate for health equity. Health professional leadership is essential to mobilise resources, build partnerships and promote meaningful change in health systems.

2. Education and Training

Health professionals can also contribute by educating and training their colleagues in other countries, sharing knowledge and best practices to strengthen global health systems. The transfer of knowledge and skills is essential to build local capacity and improve the quality of care in different contexts.

3. Research and Collaboration

Participation in international research projects and collaboration with colleagues from other countries can help advance the understanding and treatment of global health problems. Collaborative research enables the sharing of data, resources and experiences, accelerating the development of innovative and effective solutions.

Conclusion

Global action and solidarity in public health are essential to address the world's most pressing health challenges. By working together and sharing resources and knowledge, countries and organisations can promote health equity and improve health outcomes for all people. International collaboration and solidarity are essential to control the spread of infectious diseases, address health crises and improve access to advanced treatments and technologies.Health professionals have a crucial role to play in this process. Their leadership and advocacy are vital in influencing global health policy and ensuring that decisions are based on ethical and human rights principles. In addition, health professionals can contribute significantly through education and training of colleagues in other countries, thereby strengthening local capacities and improving the quality of care globally. International research and collaboration are also essential. Participating in global research projects allows health professionals to share knowledge and develop innovative solutions to complex health problems. This collaboration can accelerate the development of new therapies and vaccines, and improve our understanding of diseases and their determinants. Political will is equally crucial. Governments must demonstrate a genuine commitment to global action and solidarity in public health by adequately financing health systems, investing in robust infrastructure and promoting health equity. Inclusive and equitable health policies require political leadership and a human rights-based approach, ensuring that all citizens have access to quality health services. Examples such as the COVAX initiative, the malaria control programme and the Global Alliance for Vaccines and Immunisation (Gavi) demonstrate how international solidarity and collaboration can have a significant impact on global health. These initiatives have improved access to vaccines, reduced disease incidence and saved millions of lives, underlining the importance of working together to address health challenges. Global action and solidarity in public health are thus not only essential to address today's challenges, but also to build a healthier and more equitable future for all. Health professionals, governments and international organisations must continue to collaborate and support each other, sharing resources, knowledge and experience. Only through joint and supportive efforts can we ensure that all people, everywhere in the world, have the opportunity to enjoy a healthy and fulfilling life.

CHAPTER 11

STRATEGIES FOR IMPLEMENTING THE HEALTH DECALOGUE

The "Decalogue on Health for the 21st Century: A Global Call to Action" is a comprehensive guide designed to promote a proactive and holistic approach to wellness. Effectively implementing the ten principles of the Decalogue requires clear strategies, intersectoral collaboration and commitment at all levels of society. This chapter details practical strategies for putting each of the Decalogue principles into action, ensuring that they become a tangible and sustainable reality.

Principle 1: Integral Awareness

Strategies

1. Holistic Educational Programmes

• Develop and implement educational programmes that address physical, mental, emotional and social well-being from a holistic perspective.

• Include comprehensive health issues in school and university curricula, ensuring that students receive a complete and balanced education.

2. Awareness Campaigns

• Conduct public awareness campaigns that promote the importance of a holistic approach to health, using traditional and digital media.

• Use social media and online platforms to disseminate messages on holistic awareness, leveraging outreach and interaction with the public.

3. Continuing Education for Health Professionals

• To provide continuing education for health professionals in holistic practices and integrated approaches to care, promoting patient-centred care and the patient's environment.

• Encourage participation in workshops and seminars on integral health, constantly updating the knowledge and skills of health personnel.

Principle 2: Prevention and Self-Care

Strategies

1. Promoting Healthy Lifestyles

• Develop community programmes that promote physical activity, healthy eating and the reduction of tobacco and alcohol consumption.

• Create environments that facilitate healthy living options, such as parks, fresh food markets and safe recreational spaces.

2. Prevention Education

• Implement workshops and seminars on disease prevention andself-care in communities, schools and workplaces, tailored to local needs.

• Provide accessible and understandable educational materials on preventive measures, using brochures, educational videos and mobile applications.

3. Access to Prevention Services

• Ensure that preventive services, such as vaccinations and regular medical check-ups, are available and accessible to the entire population, regardless of geographic location or economic status.

• Develop mobile health programmes that bring preventive services to rural and hard-to-reach communities.

Principle 3: Individual and Collective Empowerment

Strategies

1. Training in Self-Management of Health

• Provide training programmes that teach individuals how to manage their health effectively, including chronic disease management and self-care techniques.

• Provide tools and resources to facilitate self-management, such as mobile applications, online platforms and practical guides.

2. Promoting Community Involvement

• Establish community support networks and self-help groups that empower individuals and communities, promoting solidarity and mutual support.

• Involve the community in the planning and implementation of health programmes, ensuring that interventions are culturally relevant and effective.

3. Empowerment Policies

• Develop policies that promote patient empowerment and active participation in health decisions, including the creation of patient councils and community health committees.

• Promote transparency and accountability in health care, ensuring that patients have access to their medical information and can make informed decisions.

Principle 4: Equity and Universal Access

Strategies

1. Inclusion Policies

• Implement policies that guarantee universal access to health services, regardless of socio-economic status, ethnicity or gender.

• Promote equity in the distribution of health resources, ensuring that vulnerable populations receive the necessary support.

2. Barrier Reduction

• Identify and reduce barriers to accessing health services, such as geographical distance, lack of transport and financial barriers.

• To provide interpretation and translation services for populations with language barriers, facilitating communication and understanding.

3. Grant Programmes

• Establish subsidy and financial assistance programmes for vulnerable populations, ensuring that they can access necessary health services without facing excessive financial burdens.

• Develop solidarity-based financing mechanisms that allow for the equitable redistribution of resources in the health system.

Principle 5: Innovation and Technology in the Service of Health

Strategies

1. Integration of Advanced Technologies

• Adopt advanced technologies, such as telemedicine, to improve access to and quality of health care, especially in rural and remote areas.

• Implement health information systems that facilitate data management and evidence-based decision-making, promoting interoperability and information security.

2. Promoting Research and Innovation

• Support research and development of new medical technologies and treatments, encouraging collaboration between academic institutions, technology companies and health organisations.

• Promote the creation of health innovation hubs, where new technological solutions are developed and tested.

3. Technological Education

• Train health professionals in the use of new technologies and digital tools, ensuring that they can integrate these technologies into their daily practice.

• Educate patients on the use of technologies for self-care and health management, facilitating access to information and services through digital platforms.

Principle 6: Health Education and Literacy

Strategies

1. Health Literacy Programmes

• Develop health literacy programmes that teach people to interpret and use health information effectively, improving their ability to make informed decisions.

• Offer workshops and educational resources in communities and schools, adapting the content to the needs and literacy levels of the participants.

2. Accessible Educational Materials

• Create and distribute educational materials in multiple formats and languages, ensuring that they are accessible to all populations, including people with visual and hearing disabilities.

• Use digital media and online platforms to expand the reach of health education by offering interactive courses and resources.

3. Promotion of Continuing Education

• Promote continuing health education for all ages, from infancy to old age, integrating health education programmes at all stages of the life cycle.

• Collaborate with community and educational organisations to integrate health education into their programmes, promoting a lifelong learning approach.

Principle 7: Cross-sectoral Collaboration

Strategies

1. Partnership Formation

• Establish partnerships between different sectors, such as education, housing, transport and environment, to address the social determinants of health in a comprehensive manner.

• Create intersectoral committees to coordinate actions and share resources, ensuring a coordinated response to health problems.

2. Integrated Community Projects

• Develop community projects that involve multiple sectors in health promotion, addressing complex problems from diverse perspectives.

• Encourage active community participation in the design and implementation of these projects, ensuring that interventions are relevant and sustainable.

3. Health Impact Assessment

• Implement health impact assessments for all intersectoral policies and projects, using the results to adjust and improve interventions.

• Promote transparency and accountability in project implementation, ensuring that resources are used efficiently and effectively.

Principle 8: Sustainability and Resilience

Strategies

1. Sustainable Practices

• Promote sustainable practices in health resource management, such as energy efficiency and waste reduction.

• Encourage the adoption of renewable energy in healthcare facilities, reducing environmental impact and improving sustainability.

2. Resilience Planning

• Develop and maintain resilience plans that prepare health systems to respond to crises and disasters, ensuring continuity of essential services.

• Train health professionals in emergency management and post-disaster recovery, strengthening response and adaptive capacity.

3. International Collaboration

• Participate in international initiatives to address global health challenges, such as climate change and pandemics, by sharing knowledge and resources.

• Promote international cooperation in research and development of sustainable and resilient solutions, ensuring a coordinated global response.

Principle 9: Ethics and Human Rights

Strategies

1. Ethics training

• Provide continuing education in ethics and human rights for health professionals, ensuring that they understand and apply these principles in their daily practice.

• Develop ethical guidelines and protocols to guide clinical practice, promoting integrity and professional responsibility.

2. Non-Discrimination Policies

• Implement non-discrimination policies at all levels of the health system, ensuring equal and respectful treatment for all patients.

• Ensure that all patients are treated equally and respectfully, regardless of their origin, gender, sexual orientation or socio-economic status.

3. Privacy Protection

• Ensure that patients' medical information is kept confidential and protected in compliance with data protection regulations.

• Establish clear procedures for the handling and protection of health data, promoting trust and confidence in the health system.

Principle 10: Global Action and Solidarity

Strategies

1. Strengthening International Cooperation

• Actively participate in international health bodies and fora, promoting collaboration and knowledge sharing between countries.

• Foster cooperation and knowledge sharing between countries, ensuring a coordinated global response to health challenges.

2. Technical Assistance Programmes

• To provide technical and financial assistance to developing countries to strengthen their health systems, promoting equity and solidarity.

• Promote the transfer of technologies and good practices, ensuring that all countries can benefit from advances in health.

3. Awareness Raising and Mobilisation

• Conduct awareness-raising campaigns on the importance of global solidarity in health, fostering a culture of mutual support and cooperation.

• Mobilise civil society and non-governmental organisations to support global health initiatives, promoting active and committed participation.

Conclusion

Implementing the "Health Decalogue for the 21st Century" requires a comprehensive and coordinated approach involving all sectors of society. The strategies described in this chapter provide a practical framework for translating these principles into concrete and sustainable action. By working together and committing to these principles, we can move towards a healthier and more equitable future for all.

This new Health Decalogue represents a transformative paradigm for health for several key reasons. First, it promotes a vision of health that goes beyond the absence of disease to encompass physical, mental, emotional and social well-being. This holistic approach recognises the complexity of human well-being and the need to address all aspects of health together. In doing so, it promotes a model of care that considers the whole individual, rather than focusing solely on specific treatments.Furthermore, by prioritising prevention and self-care, the Decalogue highlights the importance of acting before diseases develop. This shift towards a proactive and preventive approach not only improves individual health, but also reduces the burden on health systems and associated costs. Health education and the promotion of healthy lifestyles are essential to empower people to take control of their well-being. The Decalogue places a strong emphasis on equity and universal access to health services, ensuring that all people, regardless of their socio-economic status, have an equal opportunity to reach their full health potential. This principle of social justice is crucial to reduce health inequalities and promote a more inclusive and fairer health system.By integrating innovation and technology into health care, the Decalogue encourages the use of modern tools to improve efficiency, quality and access to health services. Advanced technologies, such as telemedicine and health information systems, can transform the way care is delivered, especially in remote and resource-constrained areas. Promoting intersectoral collaboration recognises that health is influenced by a wide range of factors, including education, transport, housing and the environment. By fostering partnerships between different sectors, the Decalogue enables the social determinants of health to be addressed more effectively, creating environments that promote well-being. The Decalogue also highlights the importance of sustainability and resilience, ensuring that health systems can maintain and improve care over time and adapt to crises and disasters. Promoting sustainable practices and developing resilience plans are essential to protect the health of future generations and address global challenges such as climate change and pandemics. By incorporating ethical and human rights principles, the Decalogue ensures that all health-related actions respect the dignity and rights of all people. This ethical approach is fundamental to building a health system based on equity, respect and justice.Finally, the Decalogue promotes global action and solidarity, recognising that health is a shared issue that requires international cooperation. By working together and sharing resources and knowledge, we can address the world's most pressing health challenges and ensure that everyone has access to quality care. Accordingly, the "Health Decalogue for the 21st Century" establishes a new paradigm for health by integrating these fundamental principles into a practical, actionable guide. By implementing these strategies, we can transform our approach to health, promoting holistic and equitable wellbeing for all. In the following chapters, we will explore case studies and practical examples of how these strategies have been successfully implemented in different contexts, demonstrating the positive impact of coordinated and supportive action in promoting global health.

CHAPTER 12

CASE STUDIES: SUCCESSFUL MODELS OF HEALTH CARE

Analysing successful models of health care allows us to learn from practical experiences and apply them in different contexts to improve our health systems. In this chapter, we explore a number of case studies that stand out for their innovative and effective approaches to health promotion, disease prevention and health care delivery. These examples illustrate how the principles of the Decalogue for Health can be successfully implemented, offering valuable lessons and best practices.

Case Study 1: UK National Health System (NHS)

General Description

The UK's National Health Service (NHS) is one of the world's most recognised healthcare systems, renowned for its accessibility and quality. Founded in 1948, the NHS provides medical care free at the point of use, funded primarily by general taxation. This model has been instrumental in ensuring that all UK citizens have access to high quality, comprehensive healthcare, regardless of their financial situation.

Strategies and Results

1. Universal Access

The NHS guarantees universal access to all UK residents, regardless of their socio-economic status. This approach has significantly reduced financial barriers to accessing healthcare, allowing more people to receive the care they need without fear of cost. General tax funding ensures that the system is sustained in an equitable way, with those on higher incomes contributing more, ensuring that services are available to all.

2. Strong Primary Care

The NHS focuses on strong primary care, with GPs acting as the first point of contact for patients. These doctors not only provide general medical care, but also coordinate access to specialist services when needed. Effective primary care has improved health outcomes through prevention and early detection of disease. General practitioners play a crucial role in managing chronic diseases, promoting healthy lifestyles and providing preventive care such as vaccinations and screenings.

3. Integration of Services

The NHS integrates health and social services, providing coordinated, patient-centred care. This integration allows patients to receive a holistic continuum of care that addresses both their medical and social needs. For example, mental health services are closely linked with social services, ensuring that patients with mental health problems receive the social support necessary for their recovery. Coordination between different levels of care and services has improved the efficiency and quality of care, reducing duplication of effort and improving the patient experience.

4. Innovation and Technology

The NHS has implemented advanced technologies to improve care management and access. Among these innovations are electronic health records (EHRs), which allow healthcare professionals to quickly access patient information, improving continuity and quality of care. In addition, telemedicine has been a crucial tool, especially during the COVID-19 pandemic, allowing patients to consult their doctors securely and conveniently from home. These technologies have facilitated faster and more efficient care, improving the responsiveness of the health system and patient satisfaction.

Lessons learnt

The NHS model demonstrates that public funding and free access have been effective in removing financial barriers, allowing more people to receive care without worrying about costs. A robust primary care system is crucial for the prevention and early management of disease, reducing the burden on hospital services and improving long-term health outcomes. In addition, coordination between health and social services improves patient outcomes and system efficiency, ensuring that care is comprehensive and focused on individual needs. The adoption of advanced technologies has significantly improved care management and access, demonstrating that innovation can play a key role in modernising and improving health systems.

Case Study 2: Costa Rican Health System

General Description

Costa Rica is recognised for its high quality health system and excellent health outcomes, despite being a middle-income country. The country has achieved universal health coverage through a social security system financed by employee and employer contributions, supplemented by government funds. This model has allowed Costa Rica to maintain high standards of medical care and equity in access to health services, which has contributed to significant improvements in national health indicators.

Strategies and Results

1. Universal Coverage

Costa Rica offers universal health coverage through the Caja Costarricense de Seguro Social (CCSS), which operates a nationwide network of hospitals, clinics and health centres. The CCSS, known locally as "la Caja", ensures that all residents of the country have access to health care, regardless of their ability to pay. Funding for the system comes from employee and employer contributions, as well as government subsidies, allowing it to maintain a sustainable and equitable financing structure. This universal coverage has led to greater equity in access to health services, ensuring that low-income and vulnerable populations receive quality care.

2. Emphasis on Primary Care

Costa Rica's health system focuses on primary care through the Basic Teams for Integrated Health Care (EBAIS). These teams are made up of doctors, nurses, technical assistants and social workers, and are distributed throughout the country to provide preventive and primary health care. The EBAIS are responsible for a specific community, which allows them to develop an in-depth knowledge of the health needs of their population and to provide personalised care. This approach has significantly improved the early detection and management of chronic diseases, reducing the need for hospitalisations and more costly treatments.

3. Health Promotion and Prevention

Costa Rica has implemented extensive health promotion and disease prevention programmes. These programmes include national vaccination campaigns, health education in schools and communities, and specific programmes for the prevention of non-communicable diseases such as diabetes and hypertension. In addition, the country has launched initiatives to promoting healthy lifestyles, such as physical activity and a balanced diet. These initiatives have had a remarkable impact, significantly reducing the incidence of infectious and non-communicable diseases, and improving overall public health indicators.

4. Environmental Sustainability

Costa Rica's health system also integrates sustainable practices into its management. Many health facilities use renewable energy, such as solar and wind, to reduce their carbon footprint and promote environmental sustainability. In addition, the CCSS has implemented waste management and energy efficiency programmes to ensure that hospitals and clinics operate in an environmentally friendly manner. These practices not only contribute to the sustainability of the health system, but also support the country's environmental goals, improving the quality of life and well-being of the population.

Lessons learnt

Costa Rica's experience demonstrates that universal health coverage is possible even in countries with limited resources, and that it can significantly improve health equity. A strong primary health care system, centred on Basic Integrated Health Care Teams (EBAIS), is crucial for early detection and management of diseases, thus reducing the burden on hospital services. Health promotion and disease prevention strategies are essential to improve long-term health outcomes. Furthermore, integrating sustainability into health management is not only beneficial for the health system, but also for the environment, contributing to the overall well-being of the population.

Case Study 3: Community Health Initiative in Kerala, India

General Description

The state of Kerala in India is known for its achievements in public health, despite having a relatively low income level. Kerala has implemented a comprehensive community-based approach to health, achieving health indicators comparable to those of developed countries. This success is due to a combination of innovative strategies and a strong commitment to health equity.

Strategies and Results

1. Community Participation

Kerala actively involves the community in the planning and implementation of health programmes. Community participation has been key to the acceptance and effectiveness of health interventions. Local Health Committees (LSGs) consist of community members, health officials and representatives of non-governmental organisations. These committees are responsible for identifying local health needs, planning and monitoring the implementation of health programmes. This participatory structure ensures that health interventions are aligned with community needs and preferences, increasing their effectiveness and sustainability.

2. Primary Care and Education

Kerala's health system focuses on primary health care, with a strong emphasis on education and prevention. Primary Health Care Centres (PHCs) are the backbone of Kerala's health system, providing basic medical care, preventive services and health education programmes. Health education campaigns, including community talks, educational materials and radio and television programmes, have significantly improved health knowledge and practices among the population. The PHCs also carry out immunisation programmes, health check-ups, health education and health education programmes. of infectious diseases and chronic disease management, ensuring a comprehensive continuum of care.

3. Monitoring and Response System

Kerala has developed a robust surveillance and response system to monitor and prevent infectious diseases. The Integrated Disease Surveillance System (IDSP) monitors and reports data on disease outbreaks in real time. This system uses advanced technology to collect and analyse health data, enabling a rapid and effective response to disease outbreaks.
In addition, Kerala has established Rapid Response Units (RRUs) that are trained and equipped to handle public health emergencies, including natural disasters and infectious disease outbreaks.

4. Integration of Health and Social Services

Kerala integrates health and social services, providing holistic care to its citizens. Health and social welfare programmes are closely coordinated, ensuring that patients receive comprehensive support ranging from medical care to social assistance. For example, child nutrition programmes and support for breastfeeding mothers are linked with primary care services, ensuring that families receive a holistic approach to care. This integration has improved quality of life and health outcomes, particularly for the most vulnerable populations.

Lessons learnt

Kerala's approach demonstrates that involving the community in public health improves the effectiveness and sustainability of interventions. The active participation of Local Health Committees ensures that health programmes are aligned with community needs and preferences. Education and prevention are key to improving health outcomes, and Primary Health Care Centres (PHCs) play a key role in improving health outcomes. crucial role in the provision of these services. A robust surveillance and response system is essential for infectious disease control, and the integration of health and social services provides holistic care that improves citizens' quality of life.

Case Study 4: Rwanda's Health Programme

General Description

Rwanda has made important strides in public health, rebuilding its health system after the 1994 genocide. Through a combination of innovative policies, strong leadership and international cooperation, the country has managed to significantly improve access to care and health outcomes. Rwanda has implemented programmes addressing health coverage, primary care, technological innovation, and maternal and child health, transforming its health system and setting a model for other developing countries to follow.

Strategies and Results

1. Community Health Insurance Coverage

Rwanda has established a community-based health insurance system known as Mutuelles de Santé. This system provides affordable coverage to the majority of the population, including the most vulnerable. Funded through contributions from members, the government and international donors, Mutuelles de Santé has improved access to health services by significantly reducing financial barriers. Each household pays an annual premium based on their income level, ensuring that health services are accessible to all. This approach has led to health coverage of 90% of the population, increasing equity in access to health care.

2. Primary Care and Community Services

Rwanda focuses on primary health care with a system of community health workers (CHWs) who provide basic services and health education at the local level. These CHWs, who receive ongoing training, play a crucial role in providing preventive care, managing chronic diseases and promoting healthy health practices. CHWs are organised in cooperatives and supervised by the national health system, ensuring effective coverage in even the most remote rural areas. This model has improved the early detection of diseases, the follow-up of patients with chronic conditions, and the implementation of vaccination and infectious disease control programmes.

3. Innovation in Digital Health

Rwanda has adopted digital health technologies to improve care management and access to specialised services. The use of electronic health records (EHR) has enabled better management of patient information, facilitating follow-up and care coordination. In addition, telemedicine has been crucial in providing access to specialised medical care in rural areas, where the shortage of specialists is a significant challenge. The telemedicine platform connects rural health professionals with doctors in central hospitals, enabling remote consultations and improving the quality of care. These innovations have made medical care more efficient, accessible and of high quality.

4. Maternal and Child Health Programmes

Rwanda has implemented specific programmes to improve maternal and child health, a priority area given the high risk of mortality in these populations. Programmes include antenatal care, immunisation, newborn care education and postnatal follow-up. In addition, mobile clinics and outreach programmes have been established to reach women in rural and remote areas. These programmes have drastically reduced maternal and infant mortality. For example, maternal mortality rates have declined from 1,071 per 100,000 live births in 2000 to 210 per 100,000 in 2019. Immunisation has reached levels above 95 per cent for preventable diseases such as measles and polio.

Lessons learnt

Rwanda's community health insurance model demonstrates that inclusive financing systems can improve access and equity in health, even in low-income settings. Community health workers are essential for the provision of primary care and health education, and their integration into the formal health system ensures effective and comprehensive coverage. The adoption of digital technologies can significantly improve efficiency and access to health care, especially in resource-poor areas. In addition, specific programmes for maternal and child health are crucial to reduce mortality and improve health indicators in these vulnerable populations.

Conclusion

The analysis of the case studies presented reveals a range of successful strategies and approaches to improving health systems, demonstrating how different contexts can implement effective practices to achieve significant results. These examples offer valuable lessons and reflections on the importance of universal coverage, primary care, community participation, sustainability and technological innovation.The NHS in the UK stands out for its commitment to equity in access to healthcare. Public funding and free access at the point o f use remove financial barriers, enabling all people, regardless of their financial situation, to receive high quality care. Strong primary care and the integration of social services with health services ensure a holistic and patient-centred approach. The adoption of advanced technologies, such as electronic health records and telemedicine, has improved the efficiency and accessibility of services. This model teaches us that a robust, equitable and technologically advanced health system can be sustainable and effective in improving health outcomes.Costa Rica demonstrates that it is possible to achieve universal health coverage in a middle-income country through a well-managed and well-funded social security system. Primary care, with the Basic Teams for Integrated Health Care (EBAIS), is the cornerstone of the system, ensuring a continuum of preventive care. Investment in health promotion and disease prevention has significantly reduced the incidence of infectious and non-communicable diseases. In addition, the integration of sustainable practices in the health system, such as the use of renewable energy, underlines the importance of considering environmental impact in health management. This case shows us that equity, sustainability and a preventive approach are fundamental to the long-term success of health systems.Kerala provides an impressive example of how a comprehensive community approach can achieve health outcomes comparable to those in developed countries, despite economic constraints. Active community participation in the planning and implementation of health programmes ensures that interventions are relevant and sustainable. Primary care focusing on education and prevention has significantly improved health knowledge and practices among the population. A robust surveillance and response system enables effective management of infectious diseases. Integration of health and social services provides a holistic approach that improves quality of life. Kerala teaches us that community inclusion and a preventive approach are essential for success in public health.Rwanda has made remarkable progress in public health by rebuilding its post-genocide health system. The community health insurance system, Mutuelles de Santé, has improved access and equity by reducing financial barriers. Primary health care and services community health workers have improved preventive care and chronic disease management. The adoption of digital health technologies has facilitated more efficient and accessible care. Targeted programmes for maternal and child health have drastically reduced mortality in these vulnerable populations.Rwanda demonstrates that financial inclusion, technological innovation and a community-based approach are key to improving health outcomes in low-resource settings. These case studies reflect the diversity of approaches and strategies that can be adapted and applied in different contexts to improve health systems. Universal coverage, strong primary care, community participation, sustainability and technological innovation emerge as essential pillars. By learning from these experiences, we can design and implement more equitable, efficient and resilient health systems. The key is to adapt these lessons to local realities, ensuring that every community can reach its full potential for health and well-being.

CHAPTER 13

CURRENT CHALLENGES AND FUTURE HEALTH TRENDS

The health field is constantly evolving, facing a variety of current challenges and anticipating future trends that will shape healthcare in the coming decades. Understanding these challenges and trends is crucial to developing effective and sustainable strategies to improve global health and wellbeing.

Current Health Challenges

1. Population ageing

Population ageing is a global phenomenon that presents major challenges for health systems. Increasing life expectancy and declining birth rates have led to a growth in the proportion of older people in the population.

Impact

- Increase in Chronic Diseases: Increased prevalence of chronic diseases such as diabetes, heart disease and Alzheimer's disease.
- Demand for Long-Term Care: Growing need for long-term care and palliative care services.
- Pressure on Health Systems: Increased demand for health resources and services, which may put pressure on existing health systems.

Strategies

- Promotion of Healthy Ageing: Prevention and health promotion programmes aimed at the elderly population.
- Development of Long-Term Care Services: Investment in infrastructure and services for the care of older people.
- Innovation in Assistive Technology: Implementation of technologies that support the independence and care of older people.

2. Chronic and Non-Communicable Diseases

Chronic and non-communicable diseases (NCDs) such as diabetes, heart disease, cancer and chronic respiratory diseases are the leading causes of death and disability worldwide.

Impact

- Economic burden: High costs of treatment and management of chronic diseases.
- Impact on Quality of Life: Decrease in the quality of life of affected patients.

- Health inequalities: Higher prevalence in vulnerable and low-income populations.

Strategies

- Prevention and Education: Health education and prevention programmes to reduce risk factors such as smoking, poor diet and physical inactivity.
- Integrated Disease Management: Integrated care models that coordinate the management of multiple chronic diseases.
- Access to Treatment: Improving access to affordable and effective medicines and treatments.

3. Pandemics and Emerging Infectious Diseases

Pandemics and emerging infectious diseases, such as COVID- 19, represent significant threats to global health and can have devastating effects on societies and economies.

Impact

- Mortality and Morbidity: High mortality and morbidity rates.
- Disruption of Health Services: Overburdening and collapse of health systems.
- Economic and Social Impact: Economic destabilisation and negative effects on social welfare.

Strategies

- Preparedness and Response: Develop and maintain pandemic preparedness and response plans.
- Surveillance and Early Detection: Robust surveillance and early detection systems for disease outbreaks.
- Vaccination and Treatments: Development and rapid delivery of effective vaccines and treatments.

4. Health Inequalities

Health inequalities persist around the world, disproportionately affecting vulnerable and marginalised populations.

Impact

- Unfair Access to Services: Significant differences in access to and quality of health services.
- Disparate Health Outcomes: Higher rates of disease and mortality in disadvantaged

populations.

• Economic and Social Inequalities: Health inequalities reflect and exacerbate economic and social inequalities.

Strategies

• Health Equity Policies: Implementation of policies and programmes that promote health equity.

• Universal Access to Care: Ensure universal and equitable access to essential health services.

• Social Determinants of Health: Addressing the social determinants of health, such as poverty, education and the physical environment.

Future Trends in Health

1. Digitalisation and Digital Health

Digitisation and digital health are revolutionising the way healthcare is delivered and managed, with technologies such as telemedicine, wearable devices and artificial intelligence (AI) at the forefront.

Impact

• Improved Access to Care: Telemedicine and portable devices facilitate access to care, especially in rural and underserved areas.

• Personalisation of Care: AI and health data enable personalised treatments and more precise care.

• Efficiency and Effectiveness: Digitisation improves operational efficiency and clinical effectiveness.

Strategies

• Investment in Digital Health Technology: Encourage investment and adoption of digital technologies in health systems.

• Training and Education: Train health professionals in the use of digital technologies.

• Regulation and Data Security: Establish regulatory frameworks to ensure privacy and security of health data.

2. Precision Medicine

Precision medicine is based on the personalisation of medical treatment, tailoring interventions to the individual characteristics of each patient, such as genetics, environment and lifestyle.

Impact

- Effective treatments: Greater effectiveness of treatments thanks to personalisation.
- Reduced Side Effects: Reduced risk of side effects and adverse reactions.
- Innovation in Medical Research: Advances in medical research and the development of new treatments.

Strategies

- Research and Development: Promote research in genetics and molecular biology to support precision medicine.
- Data Infrastructure: Develop robust data infrastructures to enable the analysis and application of genomic information.
- Access and Equity: Ensure that advances in precision medicine are accessible and equitable for all populations.

3. Focus on Mental Health

Mental health is gaining recognition as a crucial component of overall well-being, and there is a growing focus on addressing mental and emotional disorders.

Impact

- Improved Quality of Life: Increased focus on mental health improves quality of life and overall well-being.
- Stigma Reduction: Increasing awareness and reducing the stigma associated with mental disorders.
- Integration into Primary Care: Integration of mental health into primary care and other health services.

Strategies

- Education and Public Awareness: Campaigns to increase awareness and understanding of mental health.
- Accessible Mental Health Services: Ensure access to quality mental health services.

• Training of Professionals: To train health professionals in the management of mental and emotional disorders.

4. Focus on Sustainability

Sustainability in health involves adopting practices that ensure that health systems can operate in the long term without compromising the capacity of future generations.

Impact

• Environmental Impact Reduction: Minimising the environmental impact of health services.

• Resource Efficiency: Efficient and sustainable management of health resources.

• Social and Environmental Responsibility: Increased social and environmental responsibility in health management.

Strategies

• Sustainable Health Practices: Implement sustainable practices in health facilities and operations.

• Sustainability Education: Promote sustainability education and awareness among health professionals.

• Policies and Regulations: Develop policies and regulations that promote sustainability in the health sector.

Conclusion

Addressing current challenges and harnessing future trends in health requires a proactive, innovative and collaborative approach. Population ageing, chronic diseases, pandemics and health inequalities are challenges that demand integrated and sustainable responses. At the same time, digitalisation, precision medicine, a focus on mental health and sustainability represent opportunities to transform healthcare and improve global wellbeing.From an ethical perspective, these challenges and trends raise important considerations that must be addressed to ensure equitable and fair care. Population ageing and the rise of chronic diseases require health systems to prioritise the fair distribution of resources and the accessibility of long-term care services. This means ensuring that all people, regardless of socio-economic status, have access to the care needed to maintain a good quality of life in old age.The response to pandemics and emerging infectious diseases underscores the need for equitable preparedness and response, where resources are distributed fairly and priority is given to the most vulnerable populations. Ethics in this context requires transparency, distributive justice and the protection of human rights, preventing emergency measures from perpetuating or exacerbating existing inequalities.Digitalisation and digital health, while offering great benefits, also present ethical risks related to privacy and security of health data. It is crucial to establish sound regulatory frameworks that protect patients' information and ensure that technologies are used in a fair and accessible way for all, avoiding the digital divide. Precision medicine raises questions about equitable access to advanced treatments based on genetic information. It is essential that these advances are not reserved for the few, but are accessible to all people, regardless of their economic capacity or geographic location. This requires inclusive policies that promote equity in the research and delivery of these treatments.The focus on mental health requires an ethical reflection on the stigma and discrimination that still surround mental disorders. Health systems must ensure that all individuals are treated fairly and respectfully, promoting the integration of mental health at all levels of care and ensuring that mental health services are accessible and of high quality. Finally, sustainability in health is not only about efficient resource management, but also about intergenerational responsibility. Health systems must adopt sustainable practices that protect the environment and ensure that future generations can enjoy good health. This implies ethical resource management and long-term planning that considers the environmental impact of current decisions. By adopting effective strategies and keeping up with emerging trends, health systems can continuously improve the quality of care and the well-being of populations. In the following chapters, we will explore how these strategies can be implemented in diverse contexts and how health professionals can lead the way to a healthier and more sustainable future. In doing so, we can move towards a more equitable, efficient and resilient health system, capable of meeting the challenges of the present and the future, always with a strong ethical commitment in all our actions and decisions.

CHAPTER 14

CONCLUSIONS AND RECOMMENDATIONS FOR HEALTH PROFESSIONALS

Throughout this book, we have explored several critical aspects of healthcare, from prevention and self-care to technological innovation and intersectoral collaboration. In this final chapter, we synthesise key findings and offer practical recommendations for health professionals. These recommendations are designed to guide practitioners in implementing effective and sustainable practices that promote the health and well-being of individuals and communities.

Main conclusions

1. Integrated Approach to Health Well-being is a multidimensional state that includes physical, mental, emotional and social aspects. Adopting a holistic approach to health is essential to address all these aspects in a coordinated and effective way.

2. Importance of Prevention and Self-Care Prevention and self-care are fundamental to maintaining health and preventing disease. Promoting healthy lifestyles and self-care education can significantly reduce the burden of chronic diseases and improve quality of life.

3. Empowering Individuals and Communities Individual and collective empowerment is crucial for effective health management. Informed and empowered individuals and communities can make better decisions about their well-being and actively contribute to public health.

4. Equity and Universal Access Ensuring equity and universal access to health services is essential to reducing health inequalities. Health systems must be inclusive and accessible to all, regardless of socio-economic background, ethnicity, gender or sexual orientation.

5. Innovation and Technology Innovation and technology have the potential to transform health care, improving access, efficiency and quality of health services. It is important to integrate these tools ethically and equitably into health systems.

6. Education and Health Literacy Education and health literacy empower people to manage their health effectively. Education programmes should be accessible and tailored to the needs of different populations.

7. Intersectoral Collaboration Collaboration between different sectors is vital to address the social determinants of health and promote a healthy environment. Intersectoral partnerships can significantly improve health outcomes.

8. Sustainability and Resilience Health systems must be sustainable and resilient, able to adapt to change and respond effectively to crises and disasters. Sustainability ensures that future generations can also enjoy good health.

9. Ethics and Human Rights Ethics and human rights must underpin all health practices and policies. Respect for the dignity, autonomy and equality of patients is fundamental to quality

care.

10. Global Action and Solidarity Health is a global issue that requires international cooperation and solidarity. Coordinated efforts at the global level are essential to address the most pressing health challenges and promote health equity.

Recommendations for Health Professionals

1. Adopting a Holistic Approach

• Comprehensive assessment: Conduct health assessments that consider all aspects of the patient's well-being: physical, mental, emotional and social. This involves using multidimensional assessment tools and collaborating with other professionals, such as psychologists and social workers, to obtain a complete picture of the patient's health status.

• Personalised treatments: Develop personalised treatment plans that address the specific needs of each patient. This may include the integration of complementary therapies, lifestyle adjustments and conventional treatments tailored to the patient's individual characteristics, such as genetics, preferences and social conditions.

2. Promoting Prevention and Self-Care

• Promoting Healthy Lifestyles: Educate patients about the importance of healthy eating, regular exercise and stress reduction. Organise workshops and support groups to promote healthy habits and provide accessible resources such as mobile apps and information leaflets.

• Prevention Programmes: Implement and promote prevention programmes, such as vaccination, regular check-ups and age- and risk-specific screening. Collaborate with community organisations to conduct public health campaigns and facilitate access to preventive services.

3. Empowering Patients and Communities

• Health Education: Providing continuing health and wellness education to patients and communities. Use methods interactive and participatory activities, such as workshops, seminars and online platforms, to facilitate learning and active participation.

• Community Participation: Encourage the active participation of communities in the planning and implementation of health programmes. Engage community leaders and local organisations to identify needs, design interventions and evaluate results.

4. Ensuring Equity in Health

• Inclusive Access: Ensure that health services are accessible to all people, without discrimination. Implement accessibility policies that remove physical, economic and cultural barriers, and provide interpretation services for people with language barriers.

• Attention to Vulnerable Populations: Develop specific programmes to address the needs of the most vulnerable and disadvantaged populations. This includes the creation of mobile clinics, the provision of health services in rural areas and the implementation of strategies to reduce health disparities.

5. Integrating Innovation and Technology

• Technology Training: Train health professionals in the use of advanced technologies and digital tools. Organise training courses and practical workshops on the use of telemedicine devices, health applications and electronic medical record management systems.

• Telemedicine and Digital Health: Adopt telemedicine and other digital health technologies to improve access and efficiency of care. Encourage the use of teleconsultation platforms, remote patient monitoring and health management applications to facilitate continuous and accessible care.

6. Promoting Health Literacy and Education

• Accessible Educational Materials: Develop and distribute educational materials in accessible and understandable formats for diverse populations. Use infographics, videos and interactive content to make information more accessible and engaging.

• Ongoing Educational Programmes: Implement ongoing educational programmes that address relevant and current health issues. Collaborate with schools, universities and community organisations to offer courses and workshops that promote health literacy from an early age.

7. Fostering Cross-Sectoral Collaboration

• Strategic Partnerships: Establish partnerships with other sectors, such as education, housing and transport, to address the social determinants of health. Form intersectoral committees to coordinate efforts and resources to implement integrated public health initiatives.

• Collaborative Projects: Engage in collaborative projects that promote health and wellness at the community level. Engage diverse stakeholders, including local governments, NGOs and private companies, to develop and implement community health programmes.

8. Promoting Sustainability and Resilience

• Sustainable Practices: Adopt sustainable practices in resource management and health operations. Implement recycling, energy efficiency and waste reduction policies in health facilities.

• Resilience Plans: Develop and maintain resilience plans to respond effectively to crises and disasters. Train staff in emergency management and conduct regular drills to ensure a rapid and coordinated response.

9. Adhering to Ethical Principles and Human Rights

• Ethics training: Participate in continuing education in ethics and human rights. Offer workshops and seminars on common ethical dilemmas and the application of ethical principles in daily practice.

• Fair and Equitable Practices: Ensure that all healthcare practices respect the dignity, autonomy and rights of patients. Implement non-discrimination policies and promote an environment of respect and fairness in all interactions with patients.

10. Participate in the Global Action

• International Collaboration: Participate in international health initiatives and organisations to promote equity and global solidarity. Contribute to international cooperation projects and share knowledge and resources with health professionals from other countries.

• Global Health Policy Advocacy: Advocate for health policies that promote equity and universal access globally. Collaborate with governments and international organisations to influence the formulation of health policies that benefit the most vulnerable populations.

FINAL CONCLUSION

Throughout this book, we have explored a wide range of issues crucial to health care in the 21st century, from prevention and self-care to technological innovation and intersectoral collaboration. The role of health professionals is central to moving towards a health system that is more equitable, sustainable and focused on people's holistic wellbeing. The future of health depends on our ability to adapt, innovate and collaborate. The principles of the 21st Century Health Decalogue provide a comprehensive guide for moving towards a health system that is more equitable, sustainable and focused on people's holistic well-being. Progress towards a more equitable, sustainable and innovative health system is intrinsically linked to ethical considerations. Health professionals must adhere to ethical principles that ensure respect for the dignity, autonomy and rights of patients. Equity in health is not only a practical goal but a moral mandate. Addressing inequities and ensuring universal access to health care are ethical imperatives that must guide all health actions and policies. In this sense, health professionals have a crucial role to play in leading this change, applying these principles in their daily practice and working together to build a healthier future for all. In the end, health is a shared responsibility that requires commitment and action from all sectors of society. Only through a collective effort can we achieve a world where everyone has the opportunity to reach their full potential for health and wellbeing.

REFERENCES

Baum, F., Newman, L., & Biedrzycki, K. (2014). Equity and the social determinants of health. Global Health Action, 7(1), 23496. https://doi.org/10.3402/gha.v7.23496

Berwick, D. M., Nolan, T. W., & Whittington, J. (2008). The Triple Aim: Care, health, and cost. Health Affairs, 27(3), 759-769. https://doi.org/10.1377/hlthaff.27.3.759

Bodenheimer, T., & Sinsky, C. (2014). From triple to quadruple aim: Care of the patient requires care of the provider. Annals of Family Medicine, 12(6), 573-576. https://doi.org/10.1370/afm.1713

Chokshi, D. A., & Stine, N. W. (2013). Reconsidering the politics of public health. JAMA, 310(10), 1025-1026. https://doi.org/10.1001/jama.2013.220218

Farmer, P. E., Nizeye, B., Stulac, S., & Keshavjee, S. (2006). Structural violence and clinical medicine. PLoS Medicine, 3(10), e449. https://doi.org/10.1371/journal.pmed.0030449

Frenk, J., & Moon, S. (2013). Governance challenges in global health. New England Journal of Medicine, 368(10), 936-942. https://doi.org/10.1056/NEJMra1109339

Frenk, J. (2010). The global health system: Strengthening national health systems as the next step for global progress. PLoS Medicine, 7(1), e1000089. https://doi.org/10.1371/journal.pmed.1000089

Galea, S., & Vaughan, R. D. (2018). Public health: Science, politics, and prevention. Oxford University Press.

Gostin, L. O., & Wiley, L. F. (2016). Public health law: Power, duty, restraint.

University of California Press.

Green, L. W., & Kreuter, M. W. (2005). Health program planning: An educational and ecological approach. McGraw-Hill.

Kickbusch, I., & Gleicher, D. (2012). Governance for health in the 21st century. World Health Organization.

Koplan, J. P., Bond, T. C., Merson, M. H., Reddy, K. S., Rodriguez, M. H., Sewankambo, N. K., & Wasserheit, J. N. (2009). Towards a common definition of global health. The Lancet, 373(9679), 1993-1995. https://doi.org/10.1016/S0140-6736(09)60332-9

Marmot, M., & Wilkinson, R. (Eds.) (2005). Social determinants of health.

Oxford University Press.

McMichael, A. J., Woodruff, R. E., & Hales, S. (2006). Climate change and human health: Present and future risks. The Lancet, 367(9513), 859- 869. https://doi.org/10.1016/S0140-6736(06)68079-3

Nash, D. B., Fabius, R. J., Skoufalos, A., Clarke, J. L., & Horowitz, M. R. (2016). Population health: Creating a culture of wellness. Jones & Bartlett Learning.

National Research Council (2013). U.S. health in international perspective: Shorter lives, poorer health. National Academies Press.

Rawls, J. (2001). Justice as fairness: A restatement. Harvard University Press.
Riley, W. J. (2012). Health disparities: Gaps in access, quality and affordability of medical care. Transactions of the American Clinical and Climatological Association, 123, 167-174.

Rittel, H. W. J., & Webber, M. M. (1973). Dilemmas in a general theory of planning. Policy Sciences, 4(2), 155-169. https://doi.org/10.1007/BF01405730

Sen, A. (2001). Development as freedom. Oxford University Press.

Singer, P. A., Benatar, S. R., Bernstein, M., Daar, A. S., Dickens, B. M., MacRae, S. K., & Upshur, R. E. G. (2003). Ethics and SARS: Lessons from Toronto. BMJ, 327(7427), 1342-1344.
https://doi.org/10.1136/bmj.327.7427.1342
Starfield, B., Shi, L., & Macinko, J. (2005). Contribution of primary care to health systems and health. The Milbank Quarterly, 83(3), 457-502. https://doi.org/10.1111/j.1468-0009.2005.00409.x

The Lancet Commission on Global Health (2015). Global health 2035: A world converging within a generation. The Lancet, 382(9908), 1898-1955. https://doi.org/10.1016/S0140-6736(13)62105-4

Wilkinson, R., & Marmot, M. (Eds.) (2003). Social determinants of health: The solid facts. World Health Organization.

Woolf, S. H., & Aron, L. (Eds.) (2013). The US health disadvantage relative to other high-income countries: Findings from a National Research Council/Institute of Medicine report. National Academies Press.

World Health Organization (2010). Health systems financing: The path to universal coverage. World Health Organization.

World Health Organization (2016). Framework on integrated, people-centred health services. World Health Organization.

Zwi, A. B., & Grove, N. J. (2006). Challenges to human rights: Health and conflict. The Lancet, 367(9510), 1871-1872. https://doi.org/10.1016/S0140-6736(06)68851-2

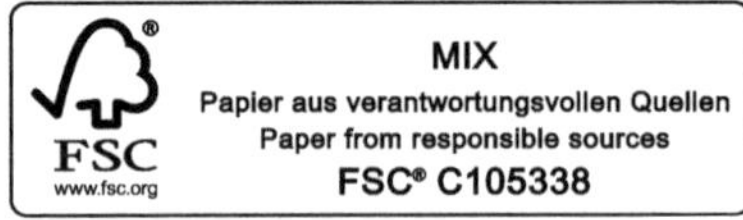

Printed by Books on Demand GmbH, Norderstedt / Germany